The Ethics of Love

Using Yoga's Timeless Wisdom to Heal Yourself, Others and the Earth

by Vimala McClure

NUCLEUS Publications

THE ETHICS OF LOVE
Using Yoga's Timeless Wisdom to Heal Yourself, Others and the Earth
by Vimala McClure

Design by Michael B. McClure

Published by NUCLEUS Publications, Rt. 2 Box 49,
Willow Springs, MO 65793. Send for a catalog.

Library of Congress Cataloging in Publication Data

McClure, Vimala Schneider, 1952—
the ethics of love: using yoga's timeless wisdom to heal yourself,
others, and the earth / by Vimala McClure.
    p.   cm.
ISBN 0-945934-08-4 : $9.00
1. Yoga. 2. Ethics, India. 3. Conduct of life. I. Title.
BJ123.Y64M33 1992
170' .954--dc20   92-28404
                                                          CIP

Table of Contents

Other books by Vimala McClure

Infant Massage: a Handbook for Loving Parents

The Tao of Motherhood

Some Still Want the Moon:
a Woman's Introduction to Tantra Yoga

Bangladesh: Rivers in a Crowded Land

Acknowledgments

The author would like to acknowledge Alcoholics Anonymous and all of the Twelve-Step Programs for their immeasurable contribution to the healing of our families, our society and our world.

This book is dedicated to my sister Madhavii, who I talk to when I need to know what is normal.

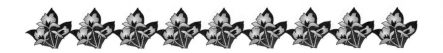

Introduction

We live in an age when human values often take a back seat to economic priorities and personal gratification. To choose a path of integrity and honesty often means to sacrifice "having it all,"— the fantasy offered by media and big business as the American Dream. We are told that only the "tough" survive—those who are willing to ignore their conscience and stretch their values in order to reach career and financial goals.

Our leaders no longer bother with a pretense of character, honor, and principle. Rather, cynicism and hypocrisy pervade our government, our schools, our corporations and even our churches, mosques, temples and synagogues. When a famous evangelist is recorded on television openly seeking the services of a prostitute, and the next day preaches the "holy gospel" to a standing ovation, something is wrong. As values have eroded, fear has grown larger and permeated our culture.

Without attention to our values in such a climate, they begin to slowly disappear. One day we find ourselves compromising our principles; we do and say things which are in opposition to what our hearts believe; we begin to feel fragmented, our self-esteem plummets, we lose the joy of living and stop feeling. We don't know how to make social and political decisions; we are afraid to take risks; we cannot teach our children what we do not know. The grief of alienating our innermost selves poisons the very cells of our bodies and eats away at our relationships, and we wonder what it's all for. Ethical principles are as old as time, but we want a fresh approach now and then. We need to re-examine human values in the light of what we've learned about ourselves.

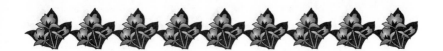

The Three Poisons: Greed, Hatred and Ignorance

The Indian sage Patanjali (who organized yoga into a spiritual discipline), spoke of the "Three Poisons" which undermine our metamorphosis from instinct-driven creatures to fully conscious human beings. As Buddhist teacher Robert Aitken points out in *The Mind of Clover:*

> ...we cannot be "holier than thou." Our society is structured on the Three Poisons of greed, hatred, and ignorance. ...Pushing heroin spiked with rat poison on a street corner is hardly Right Livelihood, but it is paradigmatic of corporations dumping carcinogenic insecticides on Latin American peasants. We are enmeshed in this cruel, acquisitive system. The tricycle your child rides may well have been manufactured by Seagram's Distilleries, or worse.

Indeed, each of us, knowingly or unknowingly, participates in many acts which go against our values each day. Becoming aware of the choices we make every day and acknowledging the pain we feel when we are unable to act upon our values keeps us moving toward the state the Sioux call the "True Human Being." Engaging in a daily dialogue with our values brings us into a state wherein the Three Poisons are constantly and consciously transmuted: greed into generosity of spirit, hatred into acceptance, ignorance into wisdom. "Just as the caterpillar suffers change, so must we," says Aitken. "The same drive that fuels the Three Poisons in the human being matures in realization of mind."

Clearly the earth is crying out for us to awaken, to become conscious of what we think, say, and do. We are capable of destroying ourselves and the earth while we allow ourselves to remain unconsciously driven by greed and hatred and to ignore the impact of our thoughts and behavior on everything around us. We are also capable of making Earth a paradise for ourselves and every animate and inanimate being which shares it with us. Very few people can confront a landslide of unconscious destruction and make a difference. But we can begin today to cultivate

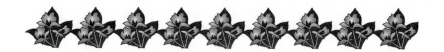

responsibility for our own little piece. We certainly cannot expect human values to resonate on a global level before we as individuals have chosen them in our own lives. Our leadership lacks a sense of unity and compassion; the conviction that we're all in this together, and our job is to make the world safe and comfortable for every being here. That kind of awareness has to begin with individuals—as Lao Tzu said, "under our feet." The only way to make changes happen is to *be* what we want to see. We may not have the power to change the minds of our world leaders. But we do have the power to change our own minds.

Yoga's code of ethics is part of what is called the Eight-Fold Path, organized by the sage Patanjali in India sometime around the second century. Other parts of this system include yoga postures and practices such as sense withdrawal, breath control, concentration, and deep meditation, all directed toward the goal of self-realization. In yoga, embracing a code of ethics is the first step toward self-realization, and an essential part of a healthy life. The reason for this is that the successful practice of meditation requires a level of mental balance and harmony wherein we are trying to bring our thoughts, words and actions into congruence. Self-realization first requires a self which is clear and true. If my heart tells me one thing and I say or do something else, the dissonance in my mind prevents me from experiencing peace. The effort to live a well-knit, honest life allows the mind to settle into calmness and clarity: to concentrate. Only then is it possible to live serenely with the confusion, pain and inconsistency of modern life, and to have the strength to confront injustice. It stands to reason that the mental peace and clarity afforded by a congruent lifestyle allows the body also to achieve a balanced state of peace and well-being, which we call health.

Behind yoga's code of ethics is an assumption that all things in the universe—animate and inanimate—are part of one eternal consciousness. Further, our goal is to merge in this conscious-

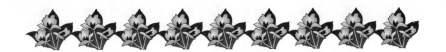

ness—known variously as the Goddess or Yahweh, the Mother, Allah or Brahma—to realize our oneness with the infinite, all-knowing Supreme. This goal isn't an event that happens in the distant future, when suddenly we "get it" and instantly become saints. It is a way of life, gradually bringing all the fragmented parts of the Self together into a whole, healthy, congruent state of being.

Mental Strength and Moral Courage: the Development of Iccha Shakti

According to yoga, the practice of value-centered living brings about a change in the very substance of our being. Those who can perceive the subtle wave-like emanations of mind are able to see a radiance—called *ojas*—in the "aura" of a person whose mind has been strengthened by a resolution to uphold personal integrity. Yoga master P.R. Sarkar says that the secret of doing effective work, of participating in effective action of any kind, is the development of Iccha Shakti, or spiritual will-power. This force of will is not ego-centered, but a strength of spirit which makes us self-confident and fearless in the face of opposition and difficulty. Each time we face a situation which violates our values and we resolve to uphold those values, our iccha shakti increases in strength, and the radiance of ojas grows. People whose iccha shakti is well-developed are powerful forces in whatever sphere they choose to live and work. These are the Davids who bring down the terrifying Three-Poisoned Goliath with one well-aimed pebble.

Our values are the foundation upon which we build wisdom, and wisdom is the only real inheritance we can leave with others when we depart. Values give our lives meaning. The expression of values which are congruent with what we know in our hearts to be right and true builds our mental strength and makes us radiant with integrity.

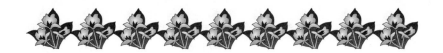

Yama and Niyama

Yoga's system of ethical precepts is divided into two parts, each with five principles. The first is *Yama* (pronounced jah-mah), which means "that which controls." The five precepts of Yama bring the Three Poisons under the control of Iccha Shakti. They are directly concerned with behavior—both that of abstinence from unhealthy thoughts, words, and actions, and the observance of healthy behaviors. The principles of Yama are about bringing our thoughts, words and behavior into awareness and consciously choosing positive, life-affirming ways of being.

Niyama (nee-yah-mah) means "self-regulation." The five principles of Niyama help us maintain a healthy, supportive environment in which we are able to grow and change.

Most people do have values. We value kindness, honesty, responsibility, clarity—our hearts beat with these values the moment we are born. But social forces have pulled us away from our hearts into our egos, which have many clever ways of rationalizing things. Love is where our hearts want to go, and generally the ego—our sense of separateness—is responsible for dragging us into its opposite: fear. Consciously choosing our values is a way to keep our minds connected with our hearts, and to heal the disease of fear which has poisoned us and our whole world. We start just by starting. "Today I'm going to observe my behavior around the issue of honesty." We bring to awareness how far our minds stray from our hearts. Awareness brings healing with it. When we become aware of how much fear and pain we are choosing, we discover our ability to choose. Then we can begin choosing love in our thoughts, in our words, and in our actions. It's not about feeling guilty, but rather a joyous journey of discovery and choice: true self-empowerment.

Ethics are only valuable to us as far as we are able to practice them in the moment-to-moment living of our lives. So it is

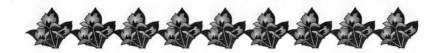

helpful to ask ourselves these questions for each of the principles to follow:

1) How does this ethic apply to me in my relationship to myself?

2) How does this ethic apply to my behavior in relationship with other beings?

3) How does this ethic apply to my social and political decisions?

PART ONE

Yama: Healthy Behavior

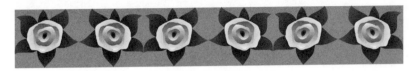

Chapter One
AHIMSA (ah-*heeng*-sah): Kindness

"Deeds of violence in our society are performed largely by those trying to establish their self-image, to defend their self-image, and to demonstrate that they, too, are significant."

—Rollo May

The essence of the practice of Ahimsa in daily life is simple kindness; kindness to ourselves, kindness to others, and compassion when making social and political choices. The word "Ahimsa" means, literally, non-harm (*a*=no, *himsa*=harm); so this kindness includes refraining from inflicting harm upon other beings.

True Ahimsa must begin with an acknowledgment of the aggressor in us—the dark, ruthless side of ourselves as human beings. Stephen Levine, in *Healing Into Life and Death*, speaks of "taking tea" with our dark side:

Most people are basically kind and gentle but haven't yet cured themselves of the reactive, injurious quality of their anger. Few have taken tea with their outrage or confusion. Most try to push it away, causing it to explode unconsciously into a world already overflowing with violence and reactivity. Few, in order to cultivate the quality of harmlessness in their lives, have taken responsibility for their anger. To take responsibility for our anger means to relate to it instead of from it. To be responsible is to be able to respond instead of having to react.

We have many opportunities to explore our destructive side; to discover and acknowledge the parts of ourselves that are capable of atrocity. Parents know the powerful forces of love which go quite beyond the soft and gentle lullaby. Threaten to harm my

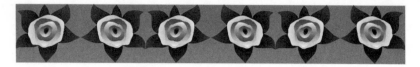

child and I can easily take your life. So much for non-violence.

But Ahimsa is not non-violence. The natural order of the universe is violent; we cannot live one minute without taking a life. We must breathe and thus destroy millions of microbes; we must eat to survive; we must protect ourselves and others from harm, sometimes by doing harm to an aggressor. The spirit of Ahimsa is the effort to bring to consciousness our impulses to do harm, and to make choices which reduce the needless harm we do. It is a way of striving to be synchronous with that which is true human nature. Rather than a "commandment," Ahimsa must be chosen with care and understanding of the motivation, the implications and consequences of one's behavior. This way of living requires constant attention, thought, choice—for it means deeply feeling the things we do (or refrain from doing) for ourselves and others. We choose what is congruent with our most honest understanding of each situation and its requirements of us.

Each of us has the capacity to harm and the capacity to bring understanding, forgiveness and kindness to meet the demons of anger, fear, and rage which cause us to harm ourselves and others. It is helpful to examine our harmful behavior with kindness toward ourselves, and then to consciously choose to practice behaviors which fuel our bodies and minds with positive energy, health and integrity.

Ahimsa in Our Personal Lives

Ahimsa means, first of all, that we take care of ourselves; as far as possible, we do no harm to our bodies. We choose not to indulge in self-destructive recreational pursuits. We feed our bodies with nutritious foods, bathe, exercise, and always try to see our bodies as beautiful, alive and precious to us. We take time to nourish our bodies every day and special time to heal our bodies when they need healing. Aggression—that tense holding-on (which we can easily recall by imagining ourselves in a traffic jam

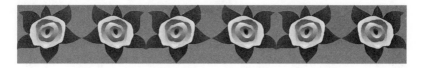

on the way to an important appointment)—sends waves of stressful impulses through our nervous systems, triggering the release of hormones which deplete our energy and undermine our immune systems. So practicing non-harm toward ourselves is more than simply refraining from harmful substances; it requires that we examine the stresses in our lives and learn how to reduce those which are unnecessary and manage those which are unavoidable.

Emotionally, Ahimsa has to do with self esteem, and with the way we turn our pain into weapons against ourselves and others. Practicing Ahimsa, we respect ourselves. Developing healthy self-respect requires that we heal the past. We try to bring to awareness experiences from childhood which injured us emotionally, experiences throughout our lives that have been harmful to us, and try to heal the damage and care for ourselves. It also means that we maintain self-respect within our relationships; that we learn how to say "No" when we need to, and how to gently but firmly let others know where our boundaries are.

Mentally, Ahimsa means that we try to keep ourselves in situations which maintain our mental peace. It means we don't beat up on ourselves; neither do we constantly demand ourselves to accomplish things of which we are incapable.

Shame is a self-destructive mental addiction which can undermine our physical, mental and emotional health and keep us from growing. It is the invisible "nitpicker" sitting on our shoulders, criticizing all that we do, berating us for what we haven't done, and telling us we're worthless. We may feel guilty or remorseful for something we did or did not do. We can choose to work through it with whomever we hurt and clean up the damage caused by our action or inaction. Behavior can be changed. But shame (which is often triggered by guilt) debilitates us. It is the feeling that we are *intrinsically* useless, irresponsible, ugly, bad, mean, etc. Shame usually results from childhood abuse. When

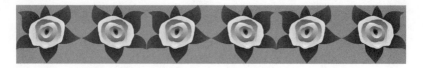

children are humiliated, blamed, degraded, criticized, disgraced, laughed at, teased, manipulated, deceived, betrayed, bullied, minimized, invalidated, and made the object of cruelty, sarcasm and scorn, shame is the poison which they internalize. While guilt involves actions which are forgivable and correctable, shame involves no hope—no way out. We can't do anything about it because it is *us*. Both guilt and shame are part of being human. However, sustaining an intimate relationship with shame uses up a tremendous amount of energy without getting anything accomplished; it depletes us and eventually transforms into resentment and anger which are then acted out in our relationships.

Often we disguise our shame and project it onto others in the form of resentment, blame, contempt, perfectionism, neglect, abandonment, and compulsive behavior. These are all ways we turn shame into a weapon in order not to feel and heal it. Practicing Ahimsa, we begin to notice shame when it arises. We can explore all the feelings that churn underneath its waves: guilt, fear, doubt, anger, aversion. With forgiveness for the pain all this is causing, we can breathe into it and name it; accept it and release it. Like the "monster in the closet" of our childhood, when the light of awareness shines upon it, shame no longer has the power to control us. It shrinks into the shadows and eventually disappears.

Ahimsa in Our Relationships

In our relationships, Ahimsa requires that we do not intentionally hurt others—groups of people as well as individuals. We observe ourselves acting out anger and resentment, being judgmental, blaming and victimizing others. Where is this behavior coming from? What triggers thoughts which make our hearts grow cold and cause us to think, speak, or act this way? With compassion toward the pain which lies beneath all of this rigidity, we can explore our thoughts and emotions and try to allow the

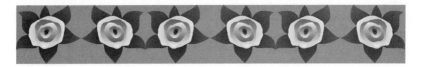

issues that cause them to come into focus.

Anger itself is not against Ahimsa; rather, it is a feeling which calls for exploration. It is the acting out of anger, without mercy for ourselves and others, which violates the spirit of Ahimsa. When we have no healthy relationship to our negative states— our rage, our fear, our frustration—we suppress them or react at ourselves and others in ways that hurt. Either only creates more of the same—not the release we seek. Stephen Levine says of anger:

> As mercy develops, we see how painful it is to be in anger and we are reminded to soften, to look gently on it as it arises. And we realize that we don't have to hellishly react, impulsively putting ourselves and the whole world out of our heart. Sensing the power of non-injury, we begin to respond to ourselves as we would to a frightened child, with a deeper kindness and care.

We can begin to explore our inner territory and discover what lies beneath our anger. Anger is like a scary mask and behind it is a frightened, hurt child. We need to find that child and heal him or her; give her the safety and love she needs. Then the mask becomes unnecessary and real communication can happen.

Ahimsa in relationships also applies to our children. We can find ways to help nurture them, guide them, and allow them to develop healthy boundaries. And we can work on reducing behaviors such as criticizing, blaming, controlling and ridiculing.

Physical and verbal abuse clearly violate the spirit of non-harm in our families. But accepting kindness as a cardinal value does not mean we never feel angry. Parents experience moments when a child brings them to the edge of sanity, when physical or verbal abuse are distinct possibilities. In that moment can grow compassion for oneself and for others' pain—and true remorse, which makes us soften and brings us closer together. Out of that moment may also grow aversion, self-hatred, intolerance for others' struggles and shame, which hardens our hearts and pushes

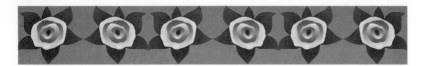

a wedge between us.

A parent who has adopted the value of Ahimsa is continuously working through feelings: exploring them and giving voice to them, finding ways to communicate them without causing damage, and learning how to guide a child with firm but supportive discipline. If we were hit and made the object of ridicule and sarcasm; if we were discounted and dismissed, it takes a conscious effort to choose other ways to discipline our own children; ways that may not be in our parenting repertoire. Acting out feelings impulsively won't work. We can find and practice ways to communicate with our children that let them know we respect them, at the same time helping them learn where our (and their) boundaries lie. Active listening, time-outs, negotiation, and choice-making are all skills which can be learned and used effectively to take the violence out of parental discipline. Nineteenth century educator Angelo Patri's advice to parents echoes that of Taoist leadership axioms:

When children try your soul, as they will; when they cause you grief, as they do; when they rouse your anger and provoke you to wrath, as is their way; when they reduce you to tears and prayer, as often happens; love them. Don't bother about anything at all until you have first made clear to yourself that your love for the child in question is holding firmly, swelling warmly in your heart. Then, whatever you do will be as nearly right as it is possible for human judgment to be right.

Not "bothering about anything at all" means that we need to withdraw, to get some time out to process our emotions and make a plan. This may mean asking someone to look after the baby for a little while or saying to a teenage daughter, "I'm really angry right now and I need some time to find my center. We will talk about this at two o'clock in the living room." We can then find someone with whom to talk through feelings and explore options.

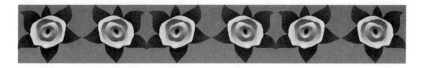

Conscious relationships are not easy, but they are simple, for they are guided from moment to moment by simple loving kindness.

Ahimsa in Our Social and Political Choices

Socially and politically, choices for Ahimsa can vary widely. Most people who practice yoga gravitate toward a vegetarian diet not only for its nutritional benefits, but because of a willingness to embrace this idea of non-harm. Naturally, if we start to think about the kinds of harm we inflict upon other beings, at some point we will think about the animals that are tortured and killed to feed us. In selecting food, the spirit of Ahimsa is to choose that in which the development of consciousness is comparatively little, judging by the capacity to express that consciousness. As my daughter says, "I don't eat things that could move off my plate by themselves if they were alive." The spirit of Ahimsa is to consider circumstances when making these decisions and make them with rationality and restraint.

Once I was sitting on the floor, talking with a young woman who had begun to meditate a year before me. She was quite intense, and was later to lose her mental balance and end up committed to a psychiatric hospital. A spider walked across the floor and I unthinkingly killed it and kept talking. She looked at me with wide eyes, shocked. "Oh! Don't do that!" she whispered. "Aren't you afraid of the karma?"

I was flustered and embarrassed, having not thought about it at all. I suddenly felt sorry that I had killed the spider without even putting my attention to it. Then I started thinking about this idea of "karma." It seemed unlikely that I would be held accountable for this is some future life, particularly when it seemed only logical that the spider's soul would be going on to bigger and better things. To refrain from killing it because of a fear for my own karma seemed not in the true spirit of Ahimsa. This little

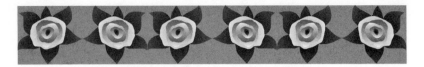

incident set off years of mulling over this precept.

I went on crushing spiders. But I was never able, after that, to unthinkingly kill anything. I have come to know myself more intimately than I did then. I know that only under the most extreme circumstances—say, protecting my child from harm or death—could I intentionally harm another person. This is a result of the combination of my history, my nature and my choice. I believe this combination is what makes for greater or lesser struggle on any ethical issue. Our histories, our deepest wounds, can make us all behave in unthinking ways which, when we are whole and healed, we would not choose. Without a keenly felt empathy and constant discrimination, without working to heal ourselves, living ethically is not possible.

A person who is gentle and accommodating by nature will have far less trouble outwardly choosing Ahimsa and living it than will someone who by nature is a warrior. However, the person with a gentle nature and unhealed wounds may strike out at the world in passive-aggressive ways, causing harm to herself and others without seeming to be responsible for it. The gentle-natured person who is whole and clear, though, and chooses Ahimsa, is a healer—a strong and clear voice of compassion and restraint.

The person with a warrior nature and unhealed wounds has a propensity for harming herself and others. Her violence is easier to spot. The unhealed warrior may find herself wishing or perpetrating pain upon those whose words or actions she opposes. The warrior nature can be put to great use, though, in the service of values and ethics, such as in the animal rights movement. The warrior who is whole and clear and who has chosen Ahimsa is a protector—a strong and clear voice of justice and courage.

Over the more than twenty years of walking a spiritual path, my growth has gradually deepened my understanding of my values. Rather than more so, this understanding has made them less automatic for me. Each day is full of tiny choices which,

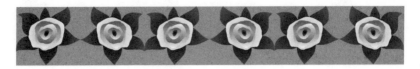

when consciously made, further my understanding and my ability to make the next choice.

Spiders have re-appeared in my life to teach me about the complexity of my choices. One day I was working in my garden, and as I bent down to inspect a flower I saw a spider web. It was perfectly round and symmetrically woven among the colorful splash of zinnias. A huge spider sat upon it. She had the most striking markings on her back. She was both beautiful and terrible. I was awestruck, and felt a tremendous respect for this creature. The thought of destroying her was barbaric—impossible. I hunkered down and watched her for a while.

A grasshopper (one among thousands which moved through the garden that year, stripping the weak plants and devouring the dead ones) sat on a leaf nearby. Suddenly, the grasshopper leapt to the very center of the web. With lightning speed, the spider pounced, wound the grasshopper into a filmy sarcophagus and hung it from the web, then returned to her previous position. I was amazed. I felt sad for the grasshopper and congratulatory toward the spider for a job well done. Each was going about its *dharma*—its innate nature—including me, whose nature it is, being human, to ponder, struggle, make mistakes, and above all, to choose.

Later that day I was walking across the yard and saw my cat pounce upon a baby rabbit, who struggled in her mouth. I strode over and told her to drop it (which startled her into doing so) and held her back as the bunny rushed off into the forest. A friend watched from a window, and opened it, yelling, "Hey, she's only following her nature!"

I laughed. "So am I!"

Recently I had yet another experience with spiders that made me realize how complex and situation-specific Ahimsa can be. There is a type of spider which is common in the Ozarks—the brown recluse. It is the most poisonous spider in the United

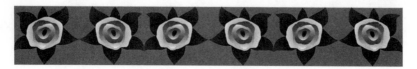

States, and it can be deadly. I was recovering from a long illness and my immune system was severely compromised. It was September, when all the spiders come out and weave their webs and have their babies. I started noticing brown recluse spiders, one after another, in my art studio. It perturbed me, but my usual way of dealing with these things is to observe the situation for a while and try to find a non-harming way to resolve it. I asked the spirit of the spiders if they would kindly find someplace else to be. I had heard that other people were able to rid their houses of unwanted insects in that manner, so I tried that first. It didn't work. More spiders came. So I killed them when I saw them. I was concerned because I knew my immune system could not tolerate very much stress and I didn't want to be bitten by one of them. But I had never been bitten by a poisonous spider before and I had never known of anyone who had been bitten by one—even among the seasoned Ozark residents—and I didn't really believe it could happen.

Then one day I found a brown recluse bite on my arm. Some might wonder if my "karma" had brought this to me. Who knows? I had a violent reaction to it which made me extremely ill for ten days. I may have been in grave danger had I been bitten again during that time. So at that point I had to make a choice: me or them. I had the exterminator come out and spray. It wasn't a solution I wanted or to which I would go immediately, not only because I value spiders in their place in nature, but also because spraying toxic chemicals is another act of harm to the environment and potentially reactive to my health. But it became apparent that it was the only rational solution. Some people might think me foolish for having waited that long. Following that incident, I no longer waited. I decided that in my environment, the spider's place was outside.

Later I learned that in Native American spirituality, the spider can symbolize creativity and letting go of fear and limitation.

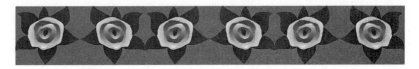

When the brown recluse spiders gathered in my art studio, and when one of them bit me, I was in the midst of a profound life change in which I was learning to let go of fears and limitations which had plagued me since childhood. I had made the decision to finally allow myself to put all of my energy into my creative work, which was in itself a frightening (but potentially exhilarating) leap for me. Being bitten by the spider was probably a coincidence. Making a symbol of it was a positive way for me to accept what the spider came to teach me. I could then release my paranoia about being bitten again and thank the spirit of the spider for reminding me to let go and commit myself to my creative work.

I was never able to come to a conclusion that spiders should always or never be destroyed. The spider has become a symbol of my relationship with nature and with the value of Ahimsa.

Living in the country, surrounded by nature and its rhythms, opportunities to think about the human's place within it come up nearly every day. This morning, as I gaze out my window at the family of deer grazing near the forest by our home, I feel a sense of wonder at their gentle beauty, and revulsion at the thought that many of my neighbors consider it fun to kill them. But if hunting were banned today, and those same neighbors' farms or jobs were compromised or lost by a proliferation of the deer population and the closing of stores, factories and agencies connected with the hunting business, would I be equally distressed?

Hunting for sport clearly violates the spirit of Ahimsa. However, we must acknowledge that attempts to legislate hunting out of existence will not work. A change of mind is required which starts with value choices on the individual level and includes efforts toward education and popularizing values which respect all life. Like many other destructive activities, hunting is a huge business upon which thousands of people's livelihood has

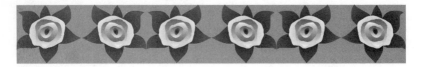

come to depend. In my area a good portion of the already depressed rural economy depends on hunting and fishing; many of my neighbors' jobs are related to hunting and so-called wildlife management. It is easy for me to agitate against hunting to save the deer; not so easy to deal compassionately with the humans who kill them. All beings deserve my respect and concern. Each choice I make has effects which ripple outward.

Given a chance, nature can balance the deer population; but in the interim a solution to the threat to crops and to the human economic problems must be found. These dilemmas are typical of the bind in which we find ourselves, having developed an economy driven by egocentric notions of human domination and control, without giving thought to long-range consequences or to values which transcend economics and politics.

Hunting as a sport has tremendous psychological power. In an article for *Animals Agenda*, Merrit Clifton suggested that in its early stages hunting is about "killing the female":

> Whether or not hunters shoot deer to demonstrate sexual potency or out of sexual frustration, in symbolic lieu of raping and killing women, there can be little doubt that as a social ritual, much hunting is all about killing the feminine in the hunter's own self. Not only are the targets male animals with the stereotypical female traits of grace and beauty, but the pursuit itself involves— indeed requires—sequestering the hunters, the men, away from female influence. Deer camp is an all-male world. Instead of cleansing themselves as women require as prelude to sexual contact, deer hunters cover themselves with "scent lures," a polite name for urine and feces. ...They wear boots indoors, curse, play poker, drink from the bottle and eat from the can—and many never actually hunt at all, getting no closer to a deer than viewing an aptly named "stag" video.

Whether it is taking the life of a sentient being or ritualistically killing a part of oneself, hunting for sport is left behind by the individual embracing Ahimsa, who feels the pain of animals

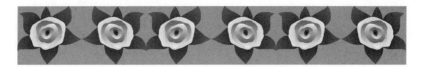

which are slaughtered because of ignorance and greed; whose journey includes uniting all aspects of one's being into a whole, compassionate Self. There is a point at which we begin to respect the life in every aspect of creation and to acknowledge the harm perpetrated on nature by human beings, whose life span has been small compared to the lifespan of the Earth. Delicate ecosystems are imperiled because we have not developed a consciousness of this value; we give no thought to what it means to harm and destroy living beings—be they trees, animals, or human beings.

When we accept Ahimsa in principle, and begin applying it in practice as far as we are able, an awareness of the rights and the intrinsic value of other living beings begins to grow. A society which accepts Ahimsa in principle will move toward the solution of the human problems its adoption presents; solutions which will also help restore the balance of nature which we have so cavalierly destroyed.

If hunting is "killing the female," the passivity of so-called nonviolence may be "killing the male." For the warrior—who courageously defends the weak and fights for truth and justice—is a part of us all, and when it is a strong part of our inner make-up, it needs an outlet. Sports and adventures which do not involve killing can be healthy outlets. Social activism, martial arts, and disaster relief work are other activities which strengthen our courage and resolve. The warrior spirit is an element of society which is needed for a vigorous, healthy balance. The story of Christ in the temple is an example of this; his righteous indignation and forceful behavior demonstrates his fearlessness in the face of exploitation, and that there are times when such action is the only healthy response. In India's epic *Mahabharata*, the Lord Krishna exhorts the Pandava brothers to take up arms against the Kaoravas, who have taken possession of the kingdom by force and are ruthlessly exploiting its people. A great battle ensues, wherein Krishna shows the warrior Arjuna that there are times when the

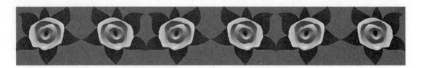

only choice is to fight, and at those times the results must be surrendered to God. These stories have both internal and external significance. Sometimes the fight is the internal commitment to find our truest selves and follow our path; to hold on to our integrity and tell the truth. Sometimes the fight must take place in the world, with words or weapons.

Some people interpret Ahimsa as refusing to participate in war. Choices range from refraining from any violent struggle to evaluating its purpose and trying to decide where the harm lies. Sometimes the lesser of evils must be chosen. For example, the harm that is done by a ruthless dictatorship to millions of innocent people may be far worse than the harm that is inflicted by an armed struggle against it. So a choice to fight, while it cannot be characterized as non-violent, may be upholding the cardinal value of Ahimsa.

Often Mahatma Gandhi's philosophy of Ahimsa is called non-violence. But an examination of the history of India's struggle for independence reveals a cunning strategy of warfare, with the weapons of forbearance on one side and the weapons of brute force on the other. The weapons of forbearance are often more powerful than the weapons of brute force, and are but one of many difficult choices faced by leaders of a resistance movement. Hundreds of thousands of people were maimed and killed in India's struggle. It cannot be characterized as a non-violent struggle, or even "passive" resistance. Rather, non-violence was a carefully and actively selected tactic with full knowledge of its implications, just as if the resistors were to face police with molotov cocktails. The people who followed Mahatma Gandhi subjected themselves (and were subjected by him) to violence in the extreme. P.R. Sarkar, in *A Guide to Human Conduct*, speaks to this issue:

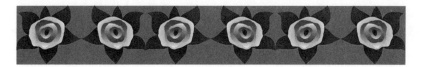

If the people of one country conquer another country by brute force, the people of the defeated nation shall use force to gain freedom. Such use of force may be crude or subtle and as a result thereof both the body and the mind of the conquerors may be wounded. When there is an application of force, it cannot be called non-violence. Is it not violence, if you hurt a man not by hand but by some indirect means? Is the boycott movement against a particular country or nation not violence? ...The mark of so-called ahimsa or non-violence on a bullet does not make the bullet non-violent.

The "direct action" of ecology groups (which some call militant, some call non-violent)—including blocking roads, sitting in small boats between whale and whaler, dismantling or disabling harmful equipment, and other "ecotage" actions to defend the environment—cannot be called non-violent. However, these actions may be ethical under certain circumstances, when choices have been systematically eliminated. Any action which may endanger life or livelihood requires a great deal of thought and communication. Gandhi insisted that communication is the element which makes any "non-violent" strategy work. Leaders must state the goals, announce intentions, and choose an action which most reduces the tendency toward violence for all parties concerned. When an action is appropriate it has great power, for it is in harmony with universal laws. Accepting Ahimsa, we work for justice without succumbing to judgmentalism; we oppose without getting locked into opposition.

Ahimsa requires conscious thought. It is not something we can decide to follow, then know what to do every day for the rest of our lives. During certain periods in our lives, we may evaluate it on a daily basis. There will be times when we are unable to find the right answer and must finally choose a course and hope the results are what we want and that we can live with them.

Abortion is such an issue, with personal as well as social and political dilemmas. Buddhist teacher Robert Aitken says:

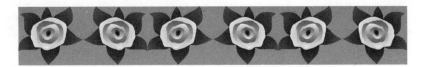

There are many personal tests of this practice [of ahimsa], from dealing with insects and mice to questions about capital punishment. Perhaps the most intimate and agonizing test is faced by the woman considering abortion. Oversimplified positions of pro-life and pro-choice do not touch the depths of her dilemma.

Ahimsa requires compassion both for the fetus, which is accepted as a living, incarnated being, and for the woman whose anguish no one else can feel. The decision to prevent birth is not an easy one, and must be made considering the suffering and pain of all within its circle.

The Buddhists have a funeral ceremony for the fetus, which brings consciousness to miscarriage or abortion and gives scope for the human need to acknowledge what has happened, to grieve and express remorse, and to send the soul of the departed on with respect and caring. Melody Ermachild wrote about one such ceremony:

As we speak, our intentions and our fates criss-cross, weaving the fabric of our complex women's lives. Outside of this room, judges on high courts make decisions while marchers hoist their picket signs. A bomb could explode in an abortion clinic. But we, as we sit, feel in our bodies what we know: She could me be, and I cannot judge her.

...I gain a deeper understanding of the meaning of what it is to be "prochoice." Choice is not control. ...Choice is a dialogue with the being who may come to life through our body. We can do no more than to bring our awareness to this sacred conversation. Something is learned from every life and every death. Choice gives us freedom, and choice asks us to accept what we have done.

In the political arena, our personal feelings about Ahimsa may require us to stand against the legalization of abortion or to fight legislation which will make it illegal. In either case, the spirit of Ahimsa is compassion for *all* beings, and to extend that compassion into acts of kindness and understanding. In choices such as

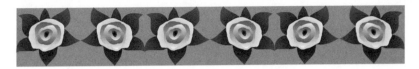

this, no one wins. To blithely dismiss the suffering of any being is contrary to Ahimsa.

It is not possible to live in the world and not do violence. But the intention to cause suffering can be explored. The value of practicing Ahimsa is in becoming conscious of the pain we cause every day. We bring to consciousness those actions which hurt ourselves and others and choose (when it is possible for us to choose) to reduce those behaviors, to refrain from those acts, and to replace them with positive, life-affirming behaviors and attitudes. Eventually the practice of Ahimsa brings us to the state of mind in which we no longer have the impulse to do harm.

Affirmation of Ahimsa

I choose to behave with kindness toward myself, others and the Earth. I choose not to, as far as it is possible, inflict pain or participate in the abuse of myself, other human beings, plants, animals, and the Earth.

Observe, Reduce, & Heal:	Practice:
Rage/resentment	Expressing anger appropriately
Impulsively reacting	Choosing to respond
Rigidity	Flexibility
Judging	Tolerance
Blaming	Accepting what is
Victimizing (mean teasing, intentionally hurting)	Giving positive encouragement
Helplessness	Taking responsibility for my life
Shame	Self-nurturing
Over-committing myself	Saying no
Allowing myself to be abused physically, mentally or emotionally	Communicating boundaries

Chapter Two
SATYA (*saht*-yah): Honesty

Oh, what a tangled web we weave when first we practice to deceive.
—William Shakespeare in *Hamlet*

Satya is speaking the truth with a spirit of kindness and living an honest life. Practicing Satya is about becoming whole and reclaiming the disowned parts of ourselves. Honesty is the only route toward wholeness, and wholeness is the real perfection.

Satya is *not* about becoming culturally perfect—becoming unreal, artificially rising above everything about us that makes us human. Perfectionism—an addiction which afflicts many of us and a web of lies which pervades our culture—is a kind of mask with attractive payoffs. It makes us feel entirely self-sufficient so we can fool ourselves into believing we do not need others (and thus do not need to be vulnerable to being hurt). It gives us a feeling of power, of being better than others ("an example") and allows us to judge, criticize, control and correct others. Perfectionism makes things black-and-white, either/or, all-or-nothing, and thus simplifies our lives and keeps us from having to deal with the anxiety of difficult choices and gray areas. It helps us avoid feeling dependent or needy, avoid trusting others, and avoid facing and accepting the unpleasant sides of ourselves.

Our culture promotes narcissism—the lie of perfectionism revisited. We are constantly assaulted by perfectionistic images on television, in movies and magazines. Women are particularly vulnerable to this attack. How many women are mentally and physically enslaved by the lure of the perfect body, the perfect face, the perfect hair, nails and teeth? How many others must fight the demons of vanity and self-battering every day because

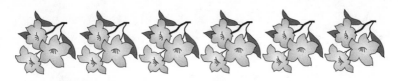

they do not possess even the *possibility* of attaining our culture's idea of perfection? I have never met a woman who has not endured this torture for at least a part of her life, if not all. And it is not "airheads" who think only about their desirability who suffer from this creativity-sapping obsession. Artistic, intelligent, powerful women who know better than to believe that physical perfection signifies their beauty suffer most from the barrage of lies from the media, from men, and from other women. There are many who profit from this self-hatred and its resultant egocentrism. We spend millions of dollars every year trying to be perfect; entire industries are dependent upon our need to hide our imperfections and mask our humanness. What would happen if we were to become totally honest; genuinely, truly ourselves? How much energy would be freed up for creative activity, for real relationships, for spiritual fulfillment?

The real perfection is becoming a human being in the same way a tree is a tree. Satya is honesty which allows us to put down the burden of superficial perfectionism and join the human race.

Satya in Our Personal Lives

In our relationship with ourselves, Satya means to be honest with ourselves. We try to understand what compels us to do and say the things we do. We look with a clear eye at our behavior and how it is a reflection of our truest selves. If we find ourselves lying, we can try to understand why. First we must address the issues that are *underlying*—what is concealed beneath. To lie is to conceal our truest selves; whether it is to make ourselves look better, to hide our imperfections and mistakes, or to try to get ahead. We can lie for years and not be aware of it. But when we shine the light of awareness on it, it becomes clear. We start becoming uncomfortable with the untruths that we project, whether through speech or through our actions or inaction.

At the same time we are becoming honest with ourselves, Satya

implies kindness. Our understanding of behavior is compassionate, so honesty about ourselves doesn't plunge us further into self-doubt, self-hatred, judgment; the thoughts that start the process of personal dishonesty. Satya is the honesty of accepting ourselves and allowing ourselves to become genuine. Kindness to ourselves means that we forgive ourselves for dishonesty and change our behavior and thoughts out of love and respect for ourselves. We can then begin to feel that we are whole human beings and that what people see is what they get. I am the same person inside as I am outside.

Anger is sometimes a kind of lie—it can often mask deeper feelings which are difficult to face. Dealing with anger in the spirit of Satya helps us go deeper. Rather than surrendering to the impulse to harm someone with words, we can spend some time discovering what pain underlies the mask of anger. Observing the tightening of our defenses, the way we direct our feelings, the moments that make up these experiences in the body and mind, we can begin to bring a different kind of energy to them. In *Healing into Life and Death*, Stephen Levine talks about bringing "a soft belly and loving kindness" into these moments. As simple as it sounds, this is the stuff of intense spiritual practice.

When my son was twelve I divorced, remarried, and moved from Colorado to Missouri. Naturally, this was a difficult time for all of us—myself, my son and daughter, my ex-husband, my husband and his son, not to mention our three cats and Chester, the dog. Each of us had challenges that pushed us up to and beyond our limits. Because of his age and temperament, the transition was hardest of all on my son. He could not reconcile himself to the move, the change of culture (from big city to rural "hillbilly" country) or the new family. After two years of grief, rage and struggle, he finally chose to move back to Denver to live with his father.

This choice was devastating to me. From the moment of their

conception, my children had been my whole world. Being a mother was the most important part of my identity, and after years of struggling with an impossibly difficult marriage, I had rejoiced in the possibility of having a real family at last. The two years of my son's unhappiness were unbearable; seeing him in so much pain because of a choice I had made was so difficult. Finally, I realized in my heart that returning to Denver was the best thing for him, and I would have to let him go. But when it happened, I fell apart. I felt as if everything that was important to me had been taken away.

I knew that keeping a "stiff upper lip" was not only unhealthy, it was simply impossible; my heart was breaking. I decided to allow myself to be in grief and to soften to it as much as I could. I noticed there was a pattern to my feelings. The unbearable sense of the loss of my child would hit my mind and heart like a hurricane. I would feel a hardness come around my heart, a kind of numbing and tightening. There would be a hard pain in my chest and stomach. Then anger would arise, and I would find myself searching for someone to blame, at whom my feelings could be unleashed; sometimes I searched for someone else—my husband came first to mind, and I would start getting furious with him. Sometimes it would be me that my mind would wish to accuse. "If only I had loved my son more," I thought. "If I had been a better mother... If I hadn't remarried..." and so on. At that moment, I would try to make my stomach soft and to bring kindness into my pain. This was one of the most difficult things I've ever done; the pain increased. It seemed to take me down into the very core of sadness. As I looked on myself and my hardness with loving kindness, the tears would start, and I would cry from the depth of my being. I had to go through this cycle many times (and not expertly) before I began to release my pain; to release my son and myself to our new life and the joys it had in store for each of us.

I discovered through this process a positive, honest approach to anger and grief, to sadness and fear, all the emotions the mind produces when it's time to let go. I discovered other benefits as well: honesty enabled me to reach out to my loved ones and gather their kindness to help me; we grew closer. It also helped my son to learn to recognize his own pain and that it is good and healthy to feel it and go through to the other side. We are closer now, than ever.

If I had not been able to explore what lay beneath my anger, I would have chosen a target and used it to further an already painful situation. Rather than strengthening my relationships, the experience of grief would have weakened them and made me bitter. Our feelings wear many faces; the spirit of Satya is to find them all and give them voices.

Satya in Our Relationships

Satya in our relationships with others means honesty and the right use of words with a spirit of benevolence. There is a difference between Satya and *rta* which means objective, brutal truth. Satya is delivering bad news with awareness of how that news will affect the person we are telling. It means protecting others who need our protection; for example, shielding an innocent person from an untrue accusation or giving support to the testimony of someone we know to be telling the truth, even when these actions are uncomfortable for us.

At one time we may be completely straightforward in our honesty, and at another time we may be reticent. Understanding the circumstances in which we find ourselves with others, there are things we may decide not to say.

Someone was visiting our family for an extended weekend and his words (when it had anything to do with children) were constantly negative. For example, one of our children didn't want to go with us to a function. He said, "She just wants to sit home

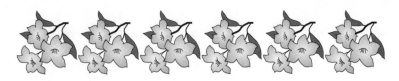

and sulk and ruin the evening for everyone." This wasn't the case at all; our child had expressed her feelings and requested not to go, but when I insisted she accompany us she came with no negative behavior, as was usual for her. This visitor would suddenly say things about the children which made us all uncomfortable, because they weren't true and they rang with such a powerful negativity that it was disturbing. I brought it up to my husband, saying it was really bothering me to hear this negativity about our children and children in general. In our home we are positive and supportive of our children, and try to always hold them in the best light and understand their stages and difficulties. At first I felt angry and my husband did too. He said he was going to say something to our friend. But as our conversation progressed it dawned on both of us that this friend had had a great deal of difficulty with his own children and stepchildren, and there were a large number of unresolved issues for which he had gotten no support in his marriage and which were painful to him. When we looked back on other times he had visited us, we remembered the first couple of days of his visit as times when negativity leaked out of him; things he kept inside came out in the supportive environment of our home. So we started to understand where this behavior was coming from, and that with continued support in a positive environment he would probably be able to understand his own behavior and his expressions would change. We decided it would be a more appropriate response for us not to say anything, but rather to give him a lot of love and support.

By the end of the visit his negativity was considerably milder. He was enjoying time with our daughter. I sensed that just being with our family was healing for him, and enabled him to open his heart and try to see things from a more positive perspective. So in that case, for us, not speaking our minds was the conscious choice. It wasn't because we were afraid of confronting him; it was truly a choice in the spirit of kindness for his welfare. Had he

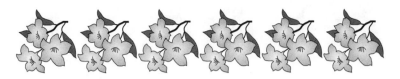

stayed with us for a long time, and had the behavior continued, our choice might have been different—the kind thing being to gently confront him.

The family gives us many opportunities to discover what Satya means to us—opportunities to make mistakes and to learn from them. With our partners it is sometimes difficult to know what level of honesty is required—particularly when a relationship is beginning. It's difficult to know how much about how we are feeling and reacting we need to say, how much confronting we should do and how much of this process needs to be kept within ourselves. The spirit of kindness is our best guide. What is the kindest thing to do in this situation, for our partner, for ourselves, and for our relationship? We need to speak the truth—even when it is not easy to face—for the sake of a relationship. We need to be honest. But we can speak with kindness. We can own our feelings—be they fear, anger, judgment—and honesty can automatically bring kindness to it and help take the "charge" out of something powerful we say to someone.

For example, my partner has done or said something that has caused me to feel a great deal of fear or rage or hurt. Perhaps what my partner said was intentional; perhaps it was unintentional. Satya requires that I first try to understand my own feelings. Perhaps what I feel is already there and my partner's words have been like a trigger, tripping the switch of rage I have brought with me from another relationship or from childhood or from a pattern that keeps repeating itself in my life that is painful to me and that I wish to change. If I can get to that—even if I can acknowledge it without fully understanding it—talking it through with my partner will be a lot easier. I can go to my partner and say, "When you said (thus and so) I felt a great deal of pain, and then I felt rage, and I still feel it. Some of this may be from my past, and I'd like to talk about that. But I also need to talk about your behavior and how you might change it so it is not

so painful for me."

Taking this a step further, we sometimes (and more often in the beginning of a relationship) need to draw our boundaries. We need to decide what we can handle and what we don't wish to handle; what we have chosen and what we have chosen not to have in our lives. Sometimes the drawing and redrawing of these boundaries can be painful. Satya requires that we be straightforward, that in the spirit of kindness for ourselves, we identify behavior that is detrimental, that invades our boundaries, that is unhealthy. In the previous example, we might not expect an overnight change, because a partner's behavior is based on his or her own history and it takes time to deal with old wounds. With patience we can heal, bring understanding to these wounds, find ways of behaving that are healthy, and practice them until the old behavior has fallen away.

But sometimes a partner resists owning his or her pain and continues behavior which is painful and triggering and which is unhealthy for the relationship. At some point I may have to go to my partner and say, "I have asked you in the past to work on changing this behavior because it is painful for me. I am working on what makes it painful for me, and I don't see anything changing from your end. I have to tell you now that I am not comfortable with accepting this behavior from you and when we get in this situation again, I will...(leave the room, point it out to you, insist we go for counseling; whatever is appropriate). I do this in the spirit of honesty, of kindness to our relationship so that a pattern is not set up of pain that goes underground and then comes out later as resentment and withholding."

Satya with our children means being as honest with them as is suitable for their age and who they are. It is not healthy to tell them everything about our lives, our inner processes, our fears, our relationships with others. But neither is it healthy to withhold ourselves from our children, to withhold the entire adult world

from them. Communicating with children involves a constant re-evaluation of what is appropriate for them. They need a gradual midwifing into their adulthood so that they can start the process of being responsible, kind and understanding people in their childhood. It starts with being able to see their parents as human beings who suffer, who are sometimes confused, who sometimes make mistakes.

Many of us grew up in households where an honest display of emotion was not allowed. Parents were not supposed to share their feelings with their children; parents were supposed to appear god-like, perfect and strong. But this withholding of feeling doesn't work to bring people closer. Many people in my generation struggle to have an honest relationship with their parents now that they are older. And they resolve to be closer to their own kids. We have begun to realize that honesty is important to close relationships; it does not reduce our power, it enhances it.

When my son was a newborn baby he was colicky and he hardly ever slept. I spent night after night awake with him. As I lost sleep I became more and more frustrated with his crying. It seemed as I grew more frustrated the crying became louder and longer. One night I found myself having fantasies of shaking him or striking him or throwing him out the window. Appalled at myself, I put him in his crib and went into the bathroom and cried. My pain at not being able to do anything for him and my frustration and exhaustion had reached its limit. As I sat there and cried, I heard his cries from the other room. I began to think that perhaps contributing to my feelings of anger was my own with-holding of my feelings from him, so that those feelings came to a point of extreme tension that could lead to battering. I suddenly understood how parents could become abusive. I decided I couldn't be any more miserable than I already was, and neither could my baby. So why not share my feelings with him? I went to him and held him in my arms and began to walk back and forth

as I had before. He cried, and I cried too. I cried out loud, I cried as loud as he cried. We walked back and forth like that for around fifteen minutes, wailing and sobbing. Then he started to calm down, and opened his eyes and looked at me. I told him how frustrated I felt, how sorry I was that I couldn't do anything that would really help him, how much I loved him, and how terrible I felt that I had abusive thoughts. I told him all this looking into his eyes, and he seemed to be listening. At that moment I stepped through a doorway into a relationship with my child that was to last a lifetime. From that point on, I listened to my child when he cried and I simply tried to be there for him in the way that I needed someone to be there for me when I cried. When I felt frustration and pain, I honestly let it show and shared it with him. This honesty has bonded us in a way that I treasure and so does he. We've been able to share our lives, and while he respects me as his mother, he also knows that he has someone with whom he is safe—even in states of anger, fear, frustration, and pain. He knows his mom isn't perfect and doesn't expect him to be perfect. He knows it's okay to say "I'm sorry," and that struggle is a part of being human.

If children are to grow up being honest, and thus benefitting themselves and the world with the power of their integrity, they need honest models. They need to see us expressing our feelings honestly, owning up to our mistakes honestly, and telling the truth in all the little ways that compose the greater Truth to which we aspire. Robert Aitken speaks of honesty as giving rise to wisdom—the ability to wisely respond to circumstances.

When a parent declares that a six-year-old child is only five in order to avoid paying an extra fare, the child learns dishonesty. If the parent acknowledges the child's correct age and buys the extra ticket, then the inherent honesty of the child is confirmed. "I'm six years old"—that's the truth.

The Insidious Nature of Dishonesty

Dishonesty is not simply lying or withholding the truth. Dishonesty is expressed in numerous ways which undermine our integrity and personal power. Observing how each of these behaviors turns up in our expressions, we can bring awareness to them and begin to replace them with positive, healthy, honest ways of being.

Denial

Denial is acting as if we don't see the truth. It can be a healthy defense. It is the first stage in the grief process, for example—a stage which helps us absorb the magnitude of a loss a little at a time. Denial is a shock absorber; it helps protect us from truths which we cannot face. But in everyday life, denial leads to disharmony within ourselves and to family dysfunction. We are taught denial in childhood when parents lie about what is happening. "Mommy's just tired." (Mommy's too drunk to stand up); "I fell down." (Daddy beat me up); "We're giving away the furniture so we can get a new set." (It's being repossessed because we're bankrupt). We thus learn that it is okay to lie about what is happening in order to fool ourselves and everyone else into believing it's always okay. The payoff is that we don't have to face the magnitude of the pain the truth sometimes brings. The problem is that denial takes a tremendous amount of energy, like constantly shoveling gravel into a bottomless pit. Underneath are the buried issues which control our lives.

We can break denial by allowing ourselves to become safe enough and strong enough to cope with the truth. Every day, in small ways, we can build strength and safety by taking care of ourselves and being honest with ourselves; by acknowledging what we cannot change and taking small steps toward changing the things we can.

Discounting

Discounting is another way to avoid the truth; it is denial made manifest in our relationships. It is a way to control other people in order to maintain a lie. The classic example in the dysfunctional family or organization is the "elephant in the living room." The family problem (alcoholism, drug addiction, religious fanaticism, abusive or criminal behavior, workaholism etc.) is like an elephant sitting in the middle of the living room. Family members sit and talk, have tea, watch television, completely ignoring the elephant. They walk around it, pretending it does not exist. When a neighbor comes in to borrow a cup of flour she exclaims, "There's an elephant in your living room!" Discounting is the dishonest way family members try to control this infraction of the "rule" of denial. They may disagree ("There is not!"), minimize ("It's just a *little* one."), defend ("So—what's it to you?"), rage ("It's none of your business! Get out of here!"), get helpless ("Oh, that—we can't do anything about it."), get righteous ("That's right, it's our elephant, so buzz off!"), make light of it ("Yes! Ha, ha! How about that?!"), try to make it normal ("Everybody has an elephant in their living room. Don't *you*?"), etc.

Other ways we discount include pretending everything is normal when it's not, teasing and ridicule, sarcasm, laughing at someone's pain, laughing at our own pain, and ignoring unhealthy situations.

Minimizing

When we are able to admit to a problem but we are unwilling to admit its depth or severity, we are minimizing. Just as there is no such thing as being sort of pregnant, there is no such thing as sort of lying, cheating or stealing. Something is either legal or illegal; it can't be "sort of" illegal. This is not all-or-nothing thinking; it is facing the truth. Often in a marriage where there

has been infidelity, one or both spouses minimize it in order to deny its impact, suppress the pain, and avoid the work it takes to heal such a huge breach of trust. Battered spouses will often say, "Well, he hit me, but not with his fist."

Excuses

Excuses and justifications, explanations and alibis help us avoid admitting we have made mistakes and avoid the work of making amends and changing our behavior. They help us avoid facing the truth and changing a situation when we are afraid of change.

Attacking

Getting righteously angry and attacking is a clever way our egos avoid the pain of facing an existing condition. It feels good to "let them have it" sometimes, and often serves the purpose of stopping someone from telling us something about ourselves we don't want to hear. Sometimes we attack out of frustration when we do not feel "heard"; it still has the effect of shutting down communication and sends a message of disrespect to the person we are attacking (which eventually rebounds). We need to express our anger or outrage, but we can find healthy ways of doing so which do not damage ourselves or have the effect of shutting out others who need to be heard.

Approval Seeking

Letting others' needs control our lives is a way we lie to ourselves and the world. When we are unable to say no and unable to say yes, we never get to tell the truth and our integrity is weakened bit by bit; our health suffers and eventually we fall apart. Approval-seeking is the lie that says, "I don't matter."

Double Messages

Satya is about clarity in thought, words and actions. Double

messages are a way to covertly and dishonestly try to control others; they create confusion, pain and rage. Often double messages are given by someone seeking the approval, service or love of another without being willing to hold up their part of the relationship. They can also come about as a result of the past interfering with the present: our present self says one thing, but our past experience makes us act out the opposite. Double binds happen when our words and actions don't match; saying, "I'm here for you," then walking out the door; saying "I need you," or "I love you," then ignoring, abandoning or abusing the other person; saying, "Tell me about it," then spacing out and not listening. Double messages discount the self and thus are destructive both to the receiver and the giver.

Broken Promises

Learning to make and keep meaningful agreements is an important part of being honest. According to Gay and Kathlyn Hendricks, authors of *Conscious Loving: The Journey Toward Co-Commitment*, making and keeping agreements is a fundamental requirement of intimacy:

> Co-commitment is made possible when two people deal with their sense of responsibility and integrity. Being alive to the full range of your feelings, speaking the truth at the deepest level of which you are capable, and learning to keep agreements: all of these actions are required to master a co-committed relationship. When these three requirements are met, the real intimacy begins to unfold. ...Once your nervous system learns to stay at a high level of aliveness and does not need to numb itself by lying, breaking agreements, and hiding feelings, the creativity starts to flow.

Keeping agreements enhances our self-esteem and increases our mental strength; breaking promises erodes both and deadens us. When an agreement must be broken or is unintentionally or unconsciously broken, Satya requires we communicate about it.

We own up to what we've done or not done and commit ourselves to exploring the issues that caused it to happen.

Conscious relationships involve a lot of choosing: choosing to tell the truth, choosing to talk about a broken promise, choosing to make amends, choosing to make agreements and choosing to keep them. Each such agreement builds trust within the relationship and integrity within the individual.

Satya in Our Social and Political Choices

Following Satya is standing up for what we believe, regardless of the consequences. As we grow and change, as we mature, our beliefs may change. What we are willing to risk for our beliefs may change, and every person has to evaluate this for him or herself. Catherine Drinker Bowen said, "I speak the truth, not so much as I would, but as much as I dare; and I dare a little more, as I grow older." I have found that as I grow older, I am learning how to speak the truth—or at least "as much as I dare"—and to accept the consequences. Growing up in an alcoholic family rife with double-binds, the truth was a confusing concept, and lying was second nature to me. While my mother spoke of the importance of honesty and telling the truth ("I can handle anything but a lie," she used to say) there was much that went on in our family that was not spoken about; lies permeated our very existence. It was many years before I began my healing and saw that my compulsion to lie was part of my childhood armor—armor that was smothering my soul. I was attracted to others who lied as a way of life, rationalizing it for good causes and justice. When I started speaking the truth, these relationships began to fall away. That was finally a risk I was willing to take.

Honesty requires a deeply felt acceptance of ourselves and the gray areas of our lives. It is not possible to attain a life free of these gray areas, these hard places, the question marks wherein the truth can hide from us. Relativity always adds a little turmoil

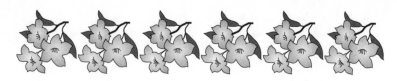

to the soup of life. The more deeply we are able to accept ourselves and others—to accept a little confusion—the more honest we can become. The more honest we become, the stronger is our integrity, and the strength to stand up for what is right when we know we must. As we pare away the little lies, the bigger ones become less tolerable. It becomes more important to speak our truth in all our relationships, in our work and home life and in our political choices. At the same time that life becomes less all-or-nothing, less black-and-white, it becomes easier to reach clarity within and act with honesty and forgiveness. The spirit of this ethic is that we think about our words and our actions and ask ourselves how honest we are being; ask ourselves, "What am I willing to risk? How courageous can I be? Is this really right?"

A great part of Satya has to do with words; with putting our feelings into words. It is speaking from the heart. It is choosing words with care and with the intention of healing—with the intention of making the world a safe place for everyone.

Affirmation of Satya

I am honest with myself today. I communicate my thoughts, feelings and beliefs with kindness in all my relationships. I choose to speak and act with integrity.

Observe, Reduce, & Heal:	Practice:
Denial	Seeing, hearing, feeling and speaking what is really going on
Discounting; sarcasm	Empowering and encouraging myself and others
Dishonesty	Honesty; appropriate self-disclosure
Approval seeking	Stating needs and feelings
Double messages	Aligning thoughts, words and actions
Breaking promises	Keeping my word

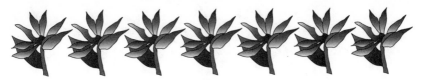

Chapter Three
Asteya (uh-*stay*-uh): Responsibility

"There are plenty of recommendations on how to get out of trouble cheaply and fast. Most of them come down to this: Deny your responsibility."

—Lyndon Johnson

Literally, Asteya means "not stealing." Simple enough. Asteya speaks directly to greed. When we choose to embrace this value in our daily lives, it starts with simply not taking what doesn't belong to us. Looking deeper, at what motivates us to steal, we come closer to the inner spirit of Asteya. Essentially, it is about withholding versus the ability to respond. We steal because we do not feel whole; when we do not feel whole we need to take from others and hold on to what we have.

Asteya in Our Personal Lives

Many people would consider Asteya a simple principle. Of course you don't steal—that's criminal. But how often are we confronted with a dilemma about withholding—money, material, information, love—and wonder what is right? When we are financially pinched and others are getting rich from cheating us, when we have deep concerns about survival, we may find ourselves justifying acts of withholding. We may not realize until later that we have diminished our innermost selves in the process. When we cheat on our income taxes, lie on an application for a loan, keep the wallet we found in the parking lot, or turn our face away from someone we love, our conscience throws up a flag: "Warning: part of your spirit has just died." Each act of straight-forward honesty builds our integrity. If we could see how these

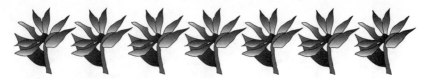

thoughts and behaviors change us—how the light of our souls increases or diminishes—our choices would be clear. But we have all kinds of clever defenses against seeing the truth—defenses which help us maintain a convenient morality. Nobody wants to be a fool or a "goody two-shoes."

In our personal lives, Asteya is about choosing to be straightforward; to speak directly, to reveal ourselves, to ask for support or help when we need it. It involves respecting our own and other people's possessions, learning how to love others unconditionally and how to help others get their needs met. We meet our obligations, return the things we borrow, and clearly state our own conditions when we make agreements. This straightforwardness—called *rjuta* in yoga—is of fundamental importance in bringing the body, mind and spirit into harmony.

Asteya in Our Relationships

In our relationships, Asteya may be broadened to include the acts of withholding with which we attempt to control ourselves and others. The extremes of over-responsibility and irresponsibility both come within the scope of Asteya.

When I am over-responsible, I try to control my environment by holding on to it; I grasp the illusion that I am the only one who knows how to do things right, that I cannot depend on others, that nobody but me cares about me and about what is important in my life. I blame myself when things go wrong, and try to compensate by pleasing everyone around me. Though it looks like I am incredibly selfless, I have actually created a world in which there is room for no one but me, me, me.

Accepting Asteya as my guide, I release control. I take 100%responsibility for my own life and feelings, and for my part of whatever relationships I am involved in. But I let go of the illusion that I know better than anyone else how to make things right. I let others live their own lives and have some of the space

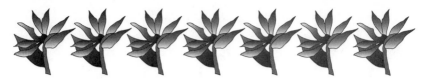

around me; I let others make their own mistakes and have their own triumphs. I release the need to be a victim of others' irresponsibility and I release the need to correct and control everyone around me. To do this, first I learn how to identify what I am feeling, to speak directly, to state my feelings and reveal myself. I take the risk of sharing my fears, asking for the help and support I want, and accepting that it's okay and I'm all right when I cannot get all that I want.

At the other extreme I create a different kind of world, but the center of that world, again, is me, me, me. I may think that I have been victimized by others and now I must focus on myself; I give myself permission to use others, ignore others' needs and avoid responsibility all in the name of "taking care of myself." At this extreme I spend most of my time getting my own needs met and I block out the needs and feelings of others around me. When threatened or confronted, I withdraw, I withhold love, and I get even.

Accepting Asteya in my life, I release my fear that others will smother me with their needs and I will disappear. I learn to listen to others and to help them get their needs met. I accept the responsibility of being interdependent with others. I learn to speak directly and ask for help, to admit it when I cannot meet my own and others' expectations, and to negotiate boundaries. I take the risk of extending myself to others, trusting that my needs will be met; and I accept that it's okay and I'm all right when I cannot get all that I want.

Asteya can also be about how we are able to receive. In his book, *Broken Toys, Broken Dreams*, Terry Kellog talks about the difficulty of receiving for people who are recovering from codependency:

Receiving can be more difficult than giving. Accepting information is more difficult than sharing information. ...The hardest thing for some of us in the

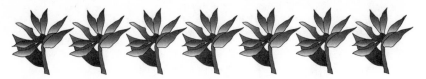

recovery process is to ask for what we need, to let others give it to us. Our shame tells us we can't depend on others. Our experience tells us we'll be disappointed. We know that we can't be vulnerable because in our vulnerability we've been hurt in the past. This is sometimes the key issue in recovery—allowing ourselves to be vulnerable, to ask and receive and when we receive, to let it be enough.

Teaching our children responsibility begins with what we do. It is important that we make our struggles known to them, that we air our difficulties and dilemmas; that we allow our children to watch and participate with us in issues regarding honesty and straightforwardness. It is important that they understand that morality is not a commandment which you follow or you don't; rather, it is a constantly evolving aspect of our humanity, and a part of us which requires attention. Our understanding of what it means to choose not to steal will change as we grow; we will make mistakes and change our minds. Living with ethics is the process of being conscious about these choices, rather than simply reacting selfishly and impulsively.

Asteya in Our Social and Political Choices

I once heard about a monk who belonged to an order which was suffering tremendous hardships financially. Donations had all but stopped and the projects they had begun—to feed the poor, build sanitary facilities in rural areas, etc.—were threatened. Some of the monks began importing things illegally and selling them on the black market in order to survive and keep the projects going. The rationale was "the ends justify the means" and "the capitalists have made this acquisitive system so they can get rich and the poor can suffer; so anything goes." They rationalized that while this activity was illegal, they didn't consider it immoral because they didn't believe in the laws that banned it. This particular young man, however, just couldn't do it. In his heart he knew that such an act would diminish him and make him ultimately

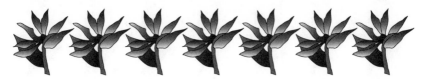

unavailable to serve humanity, so he said No. Instead, every day
he packed his battered guitar and went into the subway and sang.
He was threatened and ridiculed by the other monks, who called
him a "goody-goody" and told him he was wasting his valuable
time and humiliating himself. But it was the only thing he knew
how to do. Eventually, people put money into his guitar case and
stood by to enjoy his music. He made enough to get by, he had
time to do service, and his integrity was intact.

There is *always* another way. It may require us to humble
ourselves, or to deal with our anger and fear. It may require us to
have faith that we will be provided for. It may require us to fully
face, accept and then change the systems which exploit us. But
the first step is to draw a line, to take a stand, to say, "This is as
far as I can go in participating in exploitation and greed," and to
be willing to withstand the ridicule, censure, and scorn of others.
Without this kind of integrity, nothing can change. P.R. Sarkar
says:

When the railway is not constructed for rendering free services, non-
payment of traveling fare is theft. Think a bit; what a gentleman is he who
commits such thefts for a few rupees! Nevertheless, persons of this type indulge
in all kinds of tall talks, freely criticize leaders, accuse them of corruption and
nepotism. If their shortcoming is pointed out, they plead, "It is difficult to live
in the world with such strict morality. Those who carry on the administration
in this manner should be dealt with like this; such a theft is justified."
Missionaries or ascetics who convey a divine message or political leaders who
have the noble purpose of doing good to the country are seen in many cases
indulging in ticket-less travel. This is a daily occurrence. Bribing government
employees for evading income taxes and other taxes, or charging travelling
allowance in a higher class when the journey was actually performed in a lower
class are all nothing but cheating. It is not only theft, but also meanness.

...There are some moralists who do not want to cheat any particular individual, but do not consider anything wrong in cheating the well-to-do or the
government. Many a shopkeeper would sell adulterated commodity to the
customer but would entertain his own friends and guests with the genuine

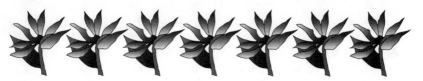

stuff. It should be remembered that all actions with such a psychological background are against Asteya.

Asteya has to do with boundaries—our personal boundaries, the boundaries in our relationships, and the boundaries of society. We all need to set limits, to choose what is healthy for us and what isn't, and to learn to respect others' choices. When we steal from others or when we withhold, we deny these limits. Boundary problems are identified by those which are too rigid or non-existent; healthy boundaries are permeable and lead to balance and a feeling of rightness.

Our society reflects what is happening in our families and personal lives with its confusion around limits and boundaries. If a poor black man steals from the convenience store, he is sent to the penitentiary; a rich white stockbroker embezzling millions pays a fine and is set free. Our immigration policy sets rigid boundaries for some and lets others in by the thousands; there is little sense to it. As Terry Kellog says:

> We invite people in, ignore their needs, give some of them a check and let them be victimized without the opportunity of integrating. We expect our sovereignty to be respected reaching way beyond our borders but we regularly violate the boundaries of others, periodically picking a small country to invade (if you're going to invade a country, a small one is the best choice).

Racism is a boundary violation, as is any expression of hatred or act of humiliation. An example of this is the controversy over the names of football teams. Native Americans have expressed dismay over names like "Redskins" and requested that these names be changed. A spokesman said that to Native Americans, the name "Redskins" is equivalent to "Niggers." No one could get away with calling a team the "Niggers." Tim Giago of the *Lakota Times*, a weekly Native American newspaper in South Dakota wrote:

48

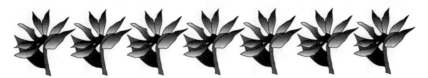

The sham rituals, such as the wearing of feathers, smoking of so-called peace pipes, beating of tomtoms, fake dances, horrendous attempts at singing Indian songs, the so-called war whoops and the painted faces, address more than the issues of racism. They are direct attacks upon the spirituality of the Indian people. ...Stop insulting the spirituality and the traditional beliefs of the Indian people by making us mascots for athletic teams. Is that asking so much of America?

The management of these teams, however, asserts that the names are a tribute to qualities such as bravery and that the fans understand this ("Aw, come on; lighten up, fellas," seems to be their position). A direct expression of protest and request for change from *the very group the teams are named for* is completely ignored—a clear violation of boundaries.

Many of the problems we face as a society have to do with boundary violations, the result of which is confusion and trauma. These include:

• Physical, emotional and sexual violence in our families, our neighborhoods, between races and nations
• Disasters such as fires, tornadoes, earthquakes, hurricanes (while we cannot control these, we can address and heal the boundary violations and their inherent trauma for those involved)
• Pollution of the air, water, and earth
• Using, torturing and killing animals for food, clothing, and testing products
• Abusing drugs, alcohol, food and sex
• An economy based on exploitation
• Spying and covert "deals" (P.R. Sarkar once said that communism as a system leads to a society of spies; capitalism to a society of thieves)
• Racism and sexism in advertising, sports and entertainment

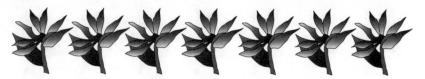

Confusion means that which is fused together; a loss of clear distinction between one thing and another. Confusion reigns when boundaries are violated. To rationalize our own lack of boundaries by pointing to the corruption in our society only brings more confusion to the issue. If we are to free ourselves from confusion, we need to start with our own lives and set some limits. We can choose not to be controlled by others. We can choose our values and choose to live by them. We can choose to say "no" and when to say "yes," and we can choose to put off decisions until we feel clear about what we want. We can learn to live with the awkwardness and discomfort it sometimes causes when we set limits. The peace we feel inside when we know who we are and can feel a healthy pride in our values is worth it.

Affirmation of Asteya
I take responsibility for every aspect of my life. I can set limits and I respect the boundaries set by others. I choose to joyfully accept my obligations to myself, others and the Earth.

Observe, Reduce, & Heal:	Practice:
Using others	Respecting others' boundaries
Theft, withholding what is due others, dishonesty with possessions	Respecting others' possessions, rules and rights
Ignoring others' needs	Helping others get their needs met
Withholding love	Loving unconditionally
Avoiding responsibility	Meeting obligations
Carrying grudges	Forgiveness
Over-responsibility	Letting go: asking for support/ help, allowing others to do for me and themselves

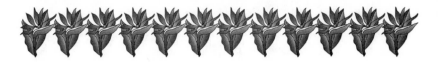

Chapter Four
Brahmacarya (brah-muh-*char*-yuh): Unity

"If we even occasionally experience our immersion within a universe that is a vast, multidimensional living organism, that experience will naturally foster a profoundly ethical posture toward the totality of life."

—Duane Elgin in *Voluntary Simplicity*

The word Brahmacarya means "to follow God." The spirit of it is to accept that a higher power permeates every atom of the universe, and there is a universal rhythm—a "flow"—that goes on beyond our comprehension and in which everything is balanced and brought to order. The spirit of unity as an ethic of everyday life is to accept that God is love and that love is the force to which we can surrender our lives.

If we think of God as a mean-spirited, spiteful giant who extracts punishment for our sins, this surrender is certainly not a good idea! But a mean-spirited God is the God we make in our fear's image. When fear grows it places limits on us and everything that comes into our world; we act with judgment and anger against ourselves and those we touch, and we place ourselves in hell. When love directs our lives—when our hearts are in charge—we act with mercy. Our world widens, becomes infused with beauty and tenderness, and we place ourselves in heaven.

We know in our hearts that God is love; we know that unconditional love is the result of something very great moving through our world. We recognize saints as those whose lives have become immersed in the energy of compassion and love for the whole universe as an expression of God—whose hearts and minds function as one, communicating that love through their words and

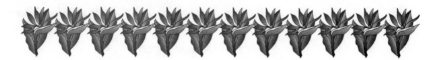

actions. Unity means the unity of our hearts and minds. It is the process of allowing love to run our lives; the unity of the individual with the Supreme. From this place, everything we come in contact with is an expression of God which has its place and its reason. It gives us the ability to distinguish between love and fear, and to choose love more often than we choose fear.

Brahmacarya in Our Personal Lives

There comes a time in our lives when something inside wakes up. Sometimes it is sudden, but more often it is a gradual stretching, slow-moving blooming-open that happens in tiny increments. It is that part of us which needs to find itself; our innermost being striving toward the perfect balance which is true humanness.

We may begin spiritual pursuits such as prayer, yoga, meditation, reading, and journal-writing. Along with these, though, if our spiritual growth is to be meaningful in our everyday lives, we need to become conscious of our moment-to-moment process. By "process" I mean our physical, mental, and emotional patterns, feelings and reactions. By observing ourselves with mindfulness, we can eventually begin to choose what we want to be and use our spiritual practices as tools to assist us. We cannot take for granted that if we meditate in such a way, if we chant so many mantras, if we hang out with spiritual people, if we go to church regularly, we will magically become what we want to be. For without applying some consciousness to the moments of our everyday lives, without attention to our own unique set of internal beliefs and reactions, our spiritual practices only serve to keep us in one place. We may not go back, but we will not go forward.

This application of consciousness to the moment is Brahmacarya. There are many ways to practice this unity of mind and heart. One way is to begin removing the masks behind which

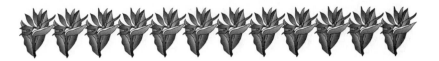

we have hidden— perhaps since childhood. This can be painful, for it means we must feel our feelings, acknowledge much about ourselves that is not ideal, speak and be the truth as it is for us. As scary as this can be it is a practice that brings us into alignment with ourselves and thus closer to God. Maria Harris, in her book *Dance of the Spirit*, likens this to taking off makeup:

It is the symbolic power of makeup that is really the issue. For cosmetics, which are probably the easiest masks to remove, are a symbol of all the masks we have learned to wear in public; masks that keep us not only from seeing ourselves, but also from being ourselves. Masks that keep us from our own aging or our own pain or our own beauty—or our own gaze.

A much more constricting and damaging mask is the false expression we so often wear: of peaceful agreement when we are in raging disagreement; of pleasure when we are actually disgusted; of distaste when we are actually delighted; of humor when we are actually repelled; of understanding when we are actually baffled. We are so out of touch with our own feelings sometimes, that we have learned to produce what we know is the expected feeling. We are so intent on pleasing others ...that we learn to fake our reactions, and when we get really good at that, we learn to stop noticing our true ones.

How often have we lied with our masks? When does the mask appear, and how? What does it feel like? We can give ourselves permission to continue wearing our masks when we need to. At the same time we can begin to allow ourselves to feel and identify what is really happening when the mask appears. Meditation can help, for it develops the concentration necessary to observe ourselves with clear eyes and it keeps our minds engaged in the truth: that we are perfect expressons of the Supreme Being and there is no need to hide or lie.

Practicing the ethic of unity, we can begin, in small ways, to risk taking off our makeup: being fully what we are in the moment, and choosing a loving way of looking at ourselves and at life. The result is serenity; a deep inner strength and peace, out of which the light of true joy can shine.

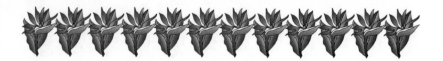

The most powerful way the practice of unity can impact our lives is that it allows us to relax. In essence, it is faith and it is surrender. It is the most powerful and empowering step we can take—to let go, lighten up, stop trying to control everything and start choosing to believe that a higher power is taking care of us and knows what it's doing. As Marianne Williamson says, "To relax, to feel the love in your heart and keep to that as your focus in every situation—that's the meaning of spiritual surrender. It changes us. We become deeper, more attractive people." We remove our masks and allow our true selves to shine.

When I was a young beginning meditator I was at a yoga ashram where several people had recently received the instruction in this lesson of unity (which, in the system of meditation I follow, involves a mantra and meditation practice to go with and assist a change in consciousness). One young man was particularly inspired about it, but hadn't yet realized what it really meant. He would stop before entering a building, close his eyes and look very holy for a minute. Then he would stop again before taking off or putting on his shoes, before eating, before getting up from the table, etc. It was amusing to watch him starting and stopping constantly. Nobody wanted to be around him because trying to interact with him was ridiculous. Before answering a question he'd close his eyes and look holy for a minute. Finally his meditation teacher saw him doing all this and took him aside, explaining to him that the practice of Brahmacarya was not an external show. He was instructed to try something more difficult: Continue your normal life, and allow yourself to feel love in every situation. When you eat, feel good about the food—enjoy its taste and texture, feel your gratitude and enjoyment and know you are cared for. When you talk to someone, relax, open up, really listen to what they have to say. When you put on your shoes, just put on your shoes! If you like your shoes, so much the better! These are the ways that a unity of heart and mind are expressed. This is

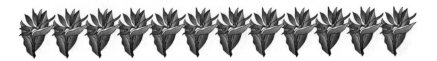

how we demonstrate that we recognize everyone and everything as an expression of God.

Brahmacarya in Our Relationships

Practicing Brahmacarya in our relationships is not an easy thing to do. It would seem that with the people we love the most it would be natural to also experience their divinity. But it is with the people we love the most that we most often engage in power struggles and righteous ego battles, and with whom we feel the most threatened and unforgiving. In our separateness, when our minds and hearts are on two different paths and we are choosing to let our minds be in charge, the ego constantly offers up fear-driven choices. Here's what the ego sounds like in my head: "It's going to be all or nothing!" "Either I get my way or he gets his way!" "Kill or be killed! Vanquish or be vanquished! Win or lose!" "Either I'm in control or I'm a victim." "Get helpless or get angry!" When I'm in a power struggle with my partner, these are the voices yelling in our heads as we try to talk to one another. What a noise! When we give in to this nonsense, we find ourselves acting out what our minds tell us. One of us becomes the bully, the other the victim, and we fight over power and control. Somebody's got to win and somebody's got to lose; somebody's going to feel guilty and somebody's going to feel righteous; grudges are nursed and our relationship is diminished.

In their book *Conscious Loving*, Gay and Kathlyn Hendricks beautifully address the issue of power struggles in a marriage, and how to get "unstuck." My partner and I didn't come across this information until we had already figured it out for ourselves; what follows is our own version—a way to help us keep the envergy moving when we are stuck in conflict and fear. These questions can be asked in any situation of conflict, whether in a marriage, between friends or business partners. They recommend both people ask and answer the following questions when the

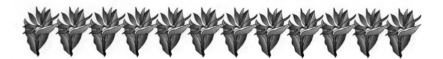

partnership is in a power struggle:

1. *How do we feel?* First we state simply and clearly the truth about our feelings: "I'm mad at you." "I'm angry." "I feel hurt." "I feel powerless." "I'm scared." With the safety of an agreement from the other person not to explode or to analyze, usually our feelings come out in layers; first anger, then sadness, then fear, then regret, and finally, love. It's important to get the feelings heard, regardless of what's "true" and what isn't. Our feelings are always true for us. At this stage we need to be like children. One partner provides the safety in which the other can childishly just "spit it out," even if it sounds like he or she is blaming the other for the conflict. If we are unable to provide this safety, we say so and take a time out to cool off, then return to listen again.

2. *What do we want?* Next, we get back to being our rational adult selves, and agree to work together to solve the conflict. We practice turning complaints into specific requests. Turn "You never listen to me" into "Will you listen to me without interrupting whileI talk about my work?"

3. *How is the past affecting the present?* What wounds might we be carrying from the past that make this so painful for us? We can explore together what we bring from childhood or previous relationships and how that might color our words and reactions now. We can try to understand what part of the conflict is repetitive and so needs our attention and healing.

4. *What are the benefits of staying stuck?* Negative behavior has secret payoffs; it helps maintain a kind of negative safety as we cling to beliefs that may not be appropriate or workable anymore. Staying in a power struggle means we don't have to change; that's a big payoff for our egos, but not much fun for our hearts and

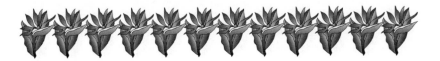

spirits, which require growth and change to stay healthy.

5. *What do we need to say?* If we're holding on to thoughts and feelings about ourselves, our partner, or the marriage that we have not expressed, they go underground and undermine the foundation. Again, we need to agree to provide safety for one another to be honest about what's going through our heads.

6. *What agreements have we broken?* Harville Hendrix, in his book *Getting the Love You Want,* says that criticism between marriage partners contains vital information for our personal growth. He says that 1) most of our partner's criticisms of us are based in truth and 2) most of our repetitive, emotional criticisms of our partner describe a disowned part of ourselves. Accepting this premise helps us to let go of our ego's struggle for control and recognize when we are breaking important agreements we have made about supporting, encouraging and listening to each other; about speaking the truth and caring for our marriage, friendship or partnership.

An important agreement my partner and I have made is not to yell at one another. We discovered that yelling is abusive in our relationship. When we cannot respond with love to each other when we're in pain, we take time out to retreat and cool off, making a date to talk at a later time. This way we do not undermine the trust and respect in our relationship, but we also do not suppress our negative feelings.

7. *How can we be of service to each other?* How can we help each other heal our wounds? How can we help each other feel supported, needed, respected, admired and cherished? How can we compromise and both get our needs met?

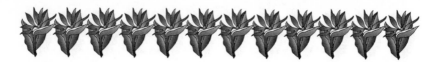

When we allow love to reign, choosing becomes a conscious moment of empowerment. When my partner and I are able to choose this way of working through things, we both get to feel good about ourselves and the growth we are choosing together. The voices of our egos may still be raging in our heads, but our love is in charge of our behavior. We can acknowledge what our minds are saying and what our hearts feel, holding firm to the truth: that we love each other completely, our intentions are good, and we wish to move into a place of support and empowerment with one another. And we find all it takes is one little moment where one of us says, "I feel (hurt, angry, enraged, attacked, belittled, helpless, neglected) and I'm willing not to be; I'm willing to see this thing in a different way." And one little moment where the other of us says, "Me too."

But what about those relationships where agreement can't be reached? In which the "me too" just won't happen? Each of us still has the capacity to choose love, to keep our hearts open even when someone else's is closed; to continue growing even when someone else doesn't seem to be. Marianne Williamson once said, "You can keep your heart open and your door locked." That is, we can choose not to allow ourselves to be abused or taken advantage of, and at the same time we can keep our hearts open and our love alive. Holding on to anger and judgment about someone diminishes us, not them. We cannot control someone else, we cannot force someone else's process. The best we can do for someone else is to try to understand where they're coming from and acknowledge what it is about their behavior that triggers our fears. We can choose not to allow fear to run our lives. Brahmacarya is about trusting love to bring us to where we want to be; to bring us into harmony with our true nature and thus to bring peace into our hearts and minds.

I believe that marriage is a place in which Brahmacarya is most called for and most tested. In its purest sense, it means faith;

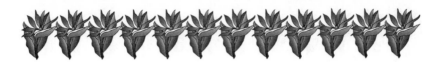

surrender. Until a marriage has been surrendered to a higher power, the commitment to it has not fully been made, and there is always a question arising as to whether it's time to call it quits. In most marriages, this surrender gradually happens over time; it must be made outwardly at a critical moment, and then it gradually "sets in." Sometimes this moment happens during the marriage ceremony, but more often it comes up after a few years of bonding, when our commitment is tested. In every marriage we are called upon to choose one another, and then choose one another again, and again, and again. Each crisis we move through deepens our commitment to the marriage itself; to the unity it represents. Without conscious choice, without conscious surrender, true commitment can never happen. In my first marriage, we unconsciously chose to sweep our issues under the rug. We couldn't face the work it would take for two such utterly different people to attain unity. We began our relationship in childhood (we were both only 16 when we were engaged) and we never re-committed to one another. Gradually our marriage dried up and became empty.

In my marriage now, there have been many re-commitments; many times when we have chosen one another again and—so far—once when we fully, consciously, outwardly surrendered our relationship to our higher power. About three years into our marriage, we had been in a power struggle for months and gotten ourselves into a situation where neither of us could "win" and if we continued, we would destroy our relationship. Finally one day we were both in so much pain we just couldn't bear it any more. We had been to marriage counseling and just couldn't find our way. We each admitted our need for help and our willingness to let go of the pain if we could just somehow be healed. We went to a favorite place and knelt down together, and we could feel so much pain—anger, hurt, bitterness and rage—vibrating the air between us. We held hands and asked, together, to be released

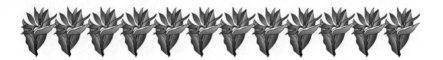

from the fear that caused us to be in pain. We asked for God to take our relationship out of our hands. And from that moment forward, things started getting better. Since then we have gotten into power struggles, fights and painful times, but there has always been a "bottom line"; a foundation of surrender to love. For us it was as if, that day, love was given supreme authority in our marriage.

For parents, a child's infancy is one of the easiest times to experience what unity feels like. I remember the hours that went by, just watching my babies and being in love with them. As children grow up and begin asserting their separateness from us, we are required to bring this choice of unity to another level. We teach our children about trusting their hearts by living from our own. And children require us to experience the pain of our separation more than just about anyone. It can be very confusing, trying to be a healthy parent when our own childhood wounded us. If we cannot find the child in us and begin to heal those wounds, we repeat whatever happened with our own parents. We project the child in us onto our own children, and react to their growth with fear.

My adolescent years were nonstop turmoil. Coming from a "broken", troubled home I was a broken, troubled child with no self esteem, no sense of personal boundaries, no trust in anything, and a lot of fear and shyness which manifested as a mask of anger and rebellion. As my own children approached adolescence fear started coming up for me again, and I was lucky to have the sense and the support to work through my own buried issues in time to separate them from the reality of who my children really are.

When I was a young teenager, I was raped on a date. I never told anyone, because I felt deeply ashamed and blamed myself. No one would believe me or help me—in those days no one talked about it, and I knew it would be assumed that I was to blame. I became a "tough" kid, started taking drugs, stealing from

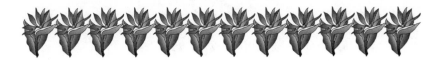

department stores, and compulsively lying. There was no safe place for me. At home, I was battered by an alcoholic stepfather and spent nearly every night crying myself to sleep.

When my daughter wanted to start dating, my first reaction was "No way!"—not because I knew it was the wrong choice, but simply out of my fears. Remembering my own pain, I expected the worst for her. We sat down one day and talked about it. I began to see how different she is from who I was; how different her experience of life and the world and relationships is from mine. I began to share some of my fears and experiences with her. "This is why I feel scared when I think about you going out with boys," I told her. I shared my story, not to scare her but to help her understand me. "I had some very painful times and I want to protect you, to help you see your choices and to support you. I need to work on seeing you for who you are, and trusting your good judgment and the self-esteem and healthy personal power you have. I hope you can work on understanding my fears and help me feel comfortable about you being safe." When both of us agree to assume love is the bottom line, there's lots of room for us both to grow, to get our needs met, and to continue feeling unity as we separate to live our own lives.

Brahmacarya in Our Social and Political Choices

When we accept Brahmacarya as a value, it becomes the foundation for many of our social and political choices. If we believe there is an underlying unity to all things, and that unity is God or Spirit, to which we surrender our lives, it changes us. We begin to question the assumptions our society makes about nearly everything. We begin to examine why we do or refrain from doing things. We begin to be concerned that, as far as possible, our choices reflect an awareness of the value we give peace and unity versus turmoil and separation. I know many people who have turned away from lucrative careers that required turmoil, stress

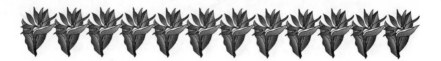

and separation so they can choose to live peacefully, joyfully and ethically. Struggle and pain will always be a part of life, but we have a choice about how that struggle will be lived—as a struggle against our deepest selves, or as a struggle to grow into wholeness. The pain we feel when we reject love—and thus reject our own spiritual nature—is much greater and more destructive than the pain we feel in the process of surrendering our egos and our fear in a leap of faith. The one makes us hard and embittered; the other makes us soft and wise. We can refuse to believe the lie that only the mean, tough, hard egoistic people survive and thrive. We can choose to believe that love is a greater power than any can pretend to be. Marianne Williamson talks about this in *A Return to Love*:

> Love is energy. It's not something we can perceive with our physical senses, perhaps, but people can usually tell you when they feel it and when they don't. Very few people feel enough love in their lives. The world has become a rather loveless place. We can hardly even imagine a world in which all of us were in love all the time, with everyone. There would be no war because we wouldn't fight. There would be no hunger because we would feed each other. There would be no environmental breakdown because we would love ourselves, our children and our planet too much to destroy it. There would be no prejudice, oppression, or violence of any kind. There would be no sorrow. There would only be peace.
>
> ...Love taken seriously is a radical outlook, a major departure from the psychological orientation that rules the world. It is threatening not because it is a small idea, but because it is so terribly huge.

Love is the basic survival requirement of every human being—even moreso than food—and it is the energy which makes everything work. In the absence of love, things begin to go awry. Our fear of the great mystery of the unseen has driven us to accept a materialistic notion of the universe as a collection of particles of lifeless matter, and consciousness as little more than the result of

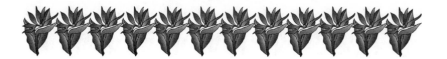

chemical reactions in the brain. In separating from nature, we separated our minds from our hearts, and began to follow the dictates of the ego in its pursuit of limitless control. Thus emerged the industrial view of reality and its self-serving philosophy, which elevates greed to the status of a social virtue. Duane Elgin, in his remarkable book *Voluntary Simplicity*, asks us to question these myths of materialism with which we were raised.

For a revitalizing society to emerge we must move beyond the industrial view of reality and human identity—we must move from greed to creative altruism, from cutthroat competition to cooperation, from "making a killing" to "earning a living," from narrow self-serving behavior to broad life-serving behavior. Instead of encouraging obliviousness to the needs of the larger world under the guise of a "natural law of the marketplace," we must encourage each individual to be more conscious of, and responsive to, the impact of his or her actions upon the rest of the world.

…Acting in a life-sensing and life-serving manner is not a spiritual platitude divorced from the hard realities of life. To the contrary, living in this way is a crucial necessity if we are to move beyond the stage of civilizational stagnation and paralysis. …If one corporate officer were to move from a life-denying and self-serving intention to that of a life-sensing and life-serving intention, that change could contribute more to meeting corporate social responsibilities than a whole new maze of government red tape and regulation. If one engineer were to make it a heartfelt intention to place the long-run well-being of the consumer and the environment above the short-run profit pursuits of the firm, that change in intention could have more impact on the design of products than, for example, a multimillion-dollar safety study funded by the federal government.

Each of us has work to do, a family to be a part of, a community in which we are—in one way or another—involved. Each of us, choosing to act in ways that affirm the value of life, of love, of unity—no matter how insignificant or tentative these actions seem to us—has tremendous power. And the more people that make this choice, the more powerful the impact on our world. We don't need to risk our lives, careers or families in this process;

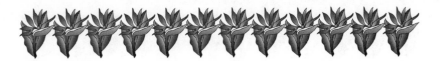

all we need to do is work on our intentions and follow our hearts. The rest will naturally unfold, bringing us and our world into harmony, into the experience of peace and unity.

Affirmation of Brahmacarya

Today I choose to believe in love. I release the fear that keeps me from feeling safe, supported, guided and cared for. I dwell in my heart.

Observe, Reduce, & Heal:	Practice:
Worrying, obsessing	Relaxing; choosing to believe I am guided and cared for by a higher power
Self-pity	Accepting myself as I am
Perfectionism	Accepting others as they are
Isolation	Open up to others
Rigid role-playing	Change appropriately; choose what I want
Superiority/inferiority	Humility
Efforts to control out of fear	Surrender to love
Fear-based beliefs	Choose to believe in love

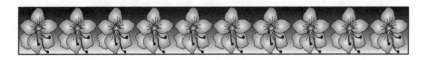

Chapter Five
Aparigraha (ah-pah-ree-*grah*-ha): Simplicity

When the Stranger says: "What is the meaning of this city?
Do you huddle close together because you love each other?"
What will you answer? "We all dwell together to make money from
each other"? or "This is a community."?

—T.S. Eliot

While Brahmacarya is concerned with the subjective experience, Aparigraha is about our objective reality; the adjustments we must all make to the world around us. Yoga's definition of simplicity is not to allow greed to dominate our thoughts and actions. It addresses our acquisitiveness, and the importance of channelling that energy toward our emotional and spiritual well-being.

Aparigraha in Our Personal Lives

In our personal lives, simplicity is aligned with honesty. To be a "simple" person is to be clear, positive, and trustworthy, without angles and agendas; without deviousness, without guile. To find simplicity, we must first begin to look clearly at our lives and what complicates them. As we bring honesty into the forefront of our values, it becomes easier to see ourselves more clearly and to know when unnecessary stresses are bringing confusion and complication into our lives.

When I moved from a large city into a rural area, I was amazed by all of the changes taking place on every level of my life. There were changes I expected and many I didn't. So much of what I took for granted in thirty-odd years of living in cities suddenly became optional. In the quiet of the countryside, I began at last

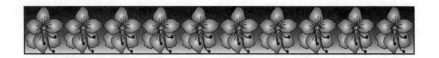

to be able to hear myself think. After a few months, I viscerally experienced having my own, original thoughts, in direct comparison to the garbled messages constantly running through my brain when I lived in the city. I became aware, as I had never been before, of the constant noise, the media jingles, news broadcasts, fads, judgments, shallowness and general negativity which had pervaded my life without my permission. I became aware of how much energy I had been using up just trying to have a life which was relatively centered.

I don't mean to say everyone needs to live in the country; of course, that is impossible and would not be everyone's choice. But to live a centered life—one which is in line with our values— it may be necessary to find some time in which to allow all of the stimulation to stop; in which to allow our own thoughts to surface. When we are able to reach our own choices through meditation and contemplation, by spending time in nature, it is much easier to find our priorities and stick to them. How much of our lives are determined by what the media impresses upon us? How many of our choices reflect a need to be politically correct, or to conform, or to gain others' approval rather than made from our hearts' conviction? How much compromise have we chosen, and how much represents an erosion of our values by all of the stimulation around us? It may be difficult—but it is not impossible—to look at our lives and choices, to figure out what our priorities are and what constitutes, for us, the necessities of life.

To choose Aparigraha is to choose an outer life that is as much in harmony with our inner values as possible. To choose simplicity is to reduce the quantity while increasing the quality. It is to face the disease of greed as it has insidiously permeated our lives and make a daily commitment to its healing.

In our personal lives, we have many opportunities to choose simplicity—not because we "should"—which implies not wanting to—but because we wish to live more compassionately.

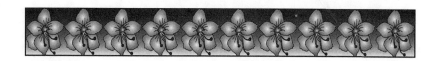

Simplicity is not self-denial, nor is it poverty; rather, it is choosing a different sort of richness. While poverty is involuntary, degrading, debilitating and engenders despair, simplicity is chosen. It is enlivening, liberating, and it engenders empowerment. Choosing to live simply is to lighten, clean up, and streamline; someone once called it "living aerodynamically." Sometimes it means spending more in the short-run with the long-run in mind. If we can afford it, it may be better to buy one expensive, well-made tool (or car, or article of clothing) that will last than to wear out and throw away several cheap substitutes. However, cost does not always insure quality, just as wealth does not insure integrity. Simplicity is about detaching ourselves from the pressure of conformity so that we can judge clearly what is appropriate for us.

Some of the choices people have made in their personal commitment to simplicity include:

• Choosing products which are ethically produced
• Participating in cooperatives—food, clothing, books, tools, repair, childcare
• Developing skills which engender self-reliance: learning how to do home and car repairs, gardening, canning, cooking, sewing, and crafts
• Participating in and developing extended family and support networks
• Choosing products which are durable, functional, beautiful and non-polluting
• Shifting diet toward vegetarian choices
• Reducing clutter through sales and give-aways
• Reducing over-all personal consumption (clothes, jewelry, cosmetics)
• Choosing work which contributes to the well-being of self and society

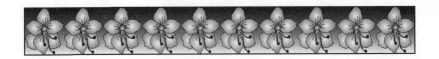

- Recycling
- Investing in small-scale projects which contribute to personal and social well-being

> It is staggering to realize how much is to be gained both for human health and for the health of the biosphere by a shift to a more plant-based diet. The historical reality is that 300 years ago North America was largely covered with luxuriant forests and tall prairie grasses. The air was clear, the waters ran pure and wildlife abounded. Since European settlers "civilized" the continent, we have cut down over half of the trees in North America, and exchanged most of them for vast fields of feedcorn, soybeans, oats, sorghum, pasture grass, hay and other forms of animal fodder. Eighty percent of the corn, oats and soybeans grown in the U.S. are not eaten by people; they are fed to livestock. We have, in effect, traded our forests for cheeseburgers.
>
> Approximately 200 million acres of land in the United States could be returned to forest with an 80 percent reduction in meat consumption. Such an immense gain would have extraordinary benefits to the whole Earth community. We would see the erosion of our topsoil halted, and our hydrological cycles renewed so that we would have more and cleaner water. Countless species of wildlife would have their habitats restored, saving them from the wave of extinction now sweeping across the planet. Because it takes 16 pounds of grain to produce a single pound of beef, but only one pound of grain to produce a pound of bread, a significant drop in meat production could mean a great deal to the world's hungry. Even a 10 percent reduction in beef consumption in the U.S. would free up enough land, water and energy to feed 60 million people—more than the number who will die of hunger and hunger-related disease on the planet this year.
>
> —**John Robbins**, author of *Diet for a New America*

Twenty years ago, when I first began to work with the value of Aparigraha in my own life, I began looking around my environment with new vision. How much of what was in my life was necessary to the quality of my life and that of the Earth? One of the first things to become clear to me was the superfluousness of a

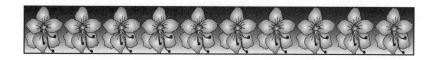

meat-centered diet. If I could survive quite healthily as a vegetarian—and the choice rested with me—why did I find it necessary to participate in the torture and murder of animals? I had to
look into my heart and ask myself if I really believed animals exist
only for their utility value to human beings. I could not find any
rationale for this position. When I could look into the eyes of an
animal—whether it be the family pet, a cow, a deer or a baby
chick—and see a sentient consciousness capable of responding,
capable of feeling pleasure and pain, I could not convince myself
that this being had no intrinsic, existential value; that it had no
right to live its life.

So I adopted a vegetarian diet and gradually brought the ethic
of simplicity into my life in other ways. It is a continuing process,
with lots of loose ends. I am not the perfect vegetarian or the
perfect animal rights consumer or the perfect ecofeminist or the
model of simplicity. I've made mistakes and taken wrong turns. I
have changed and my growth has gradually deepened my understanding of my own values. Rather than moreso, my understanding has made them less automatic for me. Each day is full of
tiny choices which, when consciously made, further my understanding and my ability to make the next choice.

Aparigraha in Our Relationships

It may at first seem that Aparigraha has little to do with our
relationships. But the value of simplicity extends into every aspect
of our lives. The clutter and accumulation of an unexamined life
often includes energy spent on relationships which have little real
value to us. To choose simplicity may mean to examine our relationships and what they mean to us. Do we spend lots of time on
many superficial relationships to the exclusion of a few strong
ones? How do we make priorities in our family relationships, our
friends, our business associates? Have we chosen and nurtured a
strong support network that will get us through troubled times?

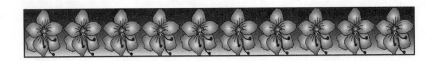

At some point we each must realize that we cannot do it all. Each choice we make is not only a choice toward something; it is also a choice away from something. When we choose to accept every invitation to parties and social gatherings, we may be choosing not to spend quiet time with our families. When we choose to chauffeur our and others' children to every school event and extracurricular activity that comes up, we may be choosing not to have any creative time for ourselves.

Aparigraha is about examining our choices and embracing our choices *not to*. We choose what we want—that which will benefit us and our world in the long run—with a clear vision of what we *don't* want. We decide what we are willing to let go and what we wish to cultivate, and we pare our lives to the simple, elegant choices which make them rich with meaning.

Aparigraha in Our Social and Political Choices

To choose simplicity is a radical move; it strikes at the very foundation of our economic structure. Our growth-oriented economy has brought us much-needed gains such as improvements in transportation, food production and distribution, and scientific research methods, and has raised our standard of living. However, it is time to reevaluate what is important to us. The growth economy is dependent upon the idea that more is always better. Thus, we have become enslaved to the rising and elusive standard of living as opposed to the quality of life.

The standard of living is measured in things and income; our quality of life is measured by people's well-being. In a growth economy one begins to push out the other. Our emphasis on economic growth undermines our sense of community and our feeling of belonging—in other words, our real sense of security. We are enslaved by the illusion that more things, more income will make us feel secure. And why not? We are deprived of the security of a community in which we have a valued place and on

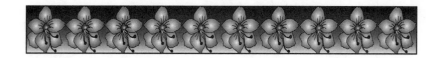

which we can depend in times of trouble.

A growth economy requires many components which undermine our real security and replace it with the false security of "getting ahead." It encourages individualism and competition over concern for others and cooperation. Our economy has reduced a sense of continuity and obligation in our families and marriages and engendered more dependence upon our individual resources and our ability to impress others. Thus, anyone who gets sick or falls behind is at risk. It has created a situation in which we must win our place in society; it is not guaranteed. And we must continually win it; the threat of losing it is always hanging over us. Without community, we must win friends, seek relationships; we must influence people. The growth economy and its large corporations require mobility, so we must continuously re-seek, re-make, re-impress people over and over, never feeling secure in our relationships. And like our place in society, ideals of competition and individualism ensure that our relationships are always threatened in some way because they tend to depend more on what we do than who we are. The pressure for growth and productivity has created a tremendous speed of change in our institutions, traditions, language, styles; we are constantly at the risk of being left out.

The ethic of growth permeates every aspect of our lives; we feel we must outgrow everything, we must get ahead, move up, move away from, not get stuck. Thus, we are continuously faced with choosing the security of a steady income over the security of long-term relationships, family and community; and our fears make us choose what our economic system wants us to choose. In fact, it lives upon our fears, and could not survive without them. Ultimately it is this system which benefits by our choices—not us. Unless everything in our lives works out perfectly (that is, we are continually successful in impressing people, we never get sick or have to take care of anyone who is sick, all our investments pay

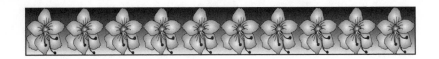

off, and nothing happens to us) we are always at risk of losing the security we have traded so dearly for. And even then—even if we make it to retirement with our income intact—we are likely to be alone in our old age, at the mercy of whatever institution we end up in (and which takes back all that closely hoarded wealth in exchange for barely maintaining our existence). Not a pretty picture. It's no wonder we try so hard not to look at it.

This obsession with growth is necessary for the huge institutions and corporations which presently operate our economic systems—and through which relatively few people profit. But it is detrimental to the fundamental well-being of people and communities. In *The Poverty of Affluence*, Paul Wachtel says, "Our overriding stress on productivity and growth and the toll it takes on our health and well being are part of a tragically unnecessary treadmill on which we run, ever more desperately, with ever more strain, committing more and more of our lives to the hopeless chase to keep up." He points out that our obsession with growth is not an inherent part of being human, nor is it inherent in a good economic system. He goes on to say:

> It is a cultural and psychological phenomenon, reflecting our present way of organizing and giving meaning to our lives… as a social phenomenon it has many of the features that in an individual would merit the term neurosis. …The heart of the notion of neurosis is the occurrence of vicious circles in peoples' behavior in which their sense of security is undermined by the very effort they make to bolster it.
>
> Inflation is part of a similar vicious circle in which the competitive, individualistic ethic we have evolved as part of our economic orientation traps us in continuing self-defeating efforts that only make matters worse. Each group tries to pull ahead of the others and almost all resist an effort to achieve a consensus of the entire national community to set limits and fix a fair level of wages and prices. This is, of course, hardly an easy thing to do; but it is impossible to do when everyone feels that he must continually have more and that it is almost his moral obligation to look out for himself and to reject as an alien ideology any commitment to the good of the community at large.

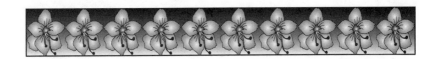

Why is it that we upgrade the minimum wage every few years, but no one dares talk about a maximum? I have never heard a public discussion of this issue. Talking about controlling the upper limits of wealth is political suicide, yet no one can comfortably live at the minimum we have established.

Everyone wants nice things and the freedom which wealth represents in our culture. But we also want to see the end of hunger and poverty. We want to ensure that everyone has a chance to live a life which is rich in significance and in which the grinding pain of struggling for daily survival is removed. Research shows that a majority of Americans place a higher priority on human values and relationships than on material values and the standard of living. But until we begin *living* this priority we will never have the courage to stand up and ask the relevant questions of those whose greed runs our lives and contributes to destroying the lives of the twenty million people living in poverty in the United States.

We must take a look at what choices we have today, and start there. We can begin to live richly and simply. We can begin to change our drive for growth from the material level to the emotional and spiritual. We can lend our support to institutions, projects, and products which support our humanness, and individuals who are engaged in life-affirming, cooperative behavior. We can build support networks which value people for who they are and which are committed to the security of the community. We can become educated and involved in our communities, and particularly in decisions toward peace, unity, cooperation, and security.

We can talk about all these issues with our children and help them to become aware of their own choices and how these choices ripple outward. In Doris Longacre's book *Living More with Less* she encourages "creative deprivation" as a way to handle simplicity with our children.

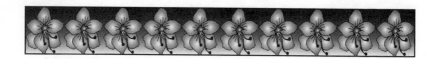

I muse on a quote by Coleman McCarthy: "To creatively deprive a child means to keep his senses and mind free of material goods that overwhelm him." It takes less than sixteen garages and their contents to choke out the qualities our children are sure to need: a gentle way of handling the earth; versatility in the face of shortage; inner provision for contentment; and more than all that, commitment to live justly in the kingdom of God.

Discussing purchases with our children (and making decisions about them together) can go a long way toward helping them feel secure and that they are participants in, rather than victims of, the family budget. Arbitrarily restricting children's material possessions out of "principle" engenders resentment. But if a child can participate in some of the larger discussions about the money coming in and going out, he or she learns a tremendous amount about living in the world, about cooperation, and about getting one's own needs met while not neglecting the needs of others. Above all, children need to know that their worth is intrinsic; it does not depend upon keeping up with the material standards of their country, their school or their neighborhood. This isn't learned simply by not allowing them to have the things other kids have. Rather, it is learned from their parents' attitudes and values as they are expressed in their words and actions in their own lives.

Affirmation of Aparigraha
Today I choose to simplify my life. I now bring my values, words and actions into harmony.

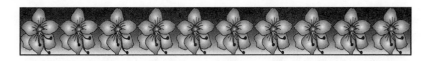

Observe, Reduce, & Heal:	Practice:
Grasping	Letting go
Denying my needs	Assessing needs, planning how to get them met
Fear-based beliefs in scarcity	Choosing to believe in love & abundance
Trying to control	Releasing control; accepting responsibility
Busy-ness; over-complicating my life & relationships	Choosing to simplify my life and make priorities
Need to accumulate things	Finding fulfillment in simplicity; building emotional and spiritual support
Discord between my values and my words and actions	Working to bring my values, words and actions into harmony

PART TWO

Niyama: Healthy Practices

The principles of Niyama help to build a lifestyle which supports the values of Yama. These are practical steps we can take to make our lives richer and more spirit-centered.

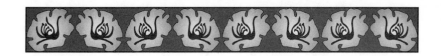

Chapter Six
SHAOCA (shah-*oh*-chah): Clarity

"The reports we get nowadays are those of men who have not gone to the scene of the accident, which is always farther inside one's head than it is convenient to penetrate without galoshes."
—E.B. White

Hanging on the wall in our office is a ceramic homily my husband and I point to when we need some reassurance about our messy lives. It says, "Creative minds are seldom tidy." We are both artists (he is a painter, I make art quilts and write books and magazine articles) and to complicate things, we have several other projects and careers going, and all at home. Without constant vigilance, some degree of organization and prioritizing, we would drown in the mess. Every space we have seems to want to become a landfill. For people who value simplicity, we've got quite a situation on our hands!

Shaoca is about getting some sort of handle on the mess, both in a practical, physical sense and in the spiritual sense. It is possible to have a clean house and a messy, complicated mind. And it is possible to have a clear mind and a messy house—but not for long.

I define Shaoca as "clarity" rather than "cleanliness" because it encompasses the whole range of behaviors around the value of being clean, clear, simple and direct. It's about cleaning the bathroom, but it's also about how our minds get cluttered with nonsense, how our world gets poisoned by the waste products of

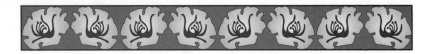

greed; and how all of these seemingly different things are connected.

Shaoca in Our Personal Lives

Cleanliness is next to Godliness. It's true. However, Godliness may not always be next to cleanliness. While a saint may look at filth and see God, if you inspect her personal life you will find the utmost care for the cleanliness of her body and surroundings, even if those surroundings are in the worst slum in the world. You will find an orderly life, an orderly mind and a sense of peace that comes through this basic value of herself. I once spent some time at Mother Teresa's baby hospital in Calcutta, India, and this principle of Shaoca was apparent everywhere I looked. Each room was simple, aesthetically decorated, and clean. All the nuns and helpers were clean and had clear, direct faces. The hundreds of babies, lined up in group cribs that stretched from one end of the room to another, were clean and their linens were fresh. It was a safe and comfortable place to be. All this came out of Mother Teresa's love for God and her respect for everything and everyone as an expression of God.

In practicing Shaoca, first of all we pay attention to our bodies and our surroundings. Do they reflect a mind at peace? We needn't cultivate the controlling personality that shrinks in horror from a little dirt and spends hours ironing towels and scrubbing the tile with a toothbrush. Rather, we can check in with our bodies and take a look at our homes, cars, property and work-places now and then and ask ourselves if they truly reflect and support our state of mind. While we can learn to accept the mess of a "work in progress," taking steps to organize our workplaces and clean up our homes empowers us. It is yet another aspect of bringing consciousness to our choices and peace to our hearts. Chinese philosopher Lao Tzu said, "He who values his body more than dominion over the empire can be given custody of the

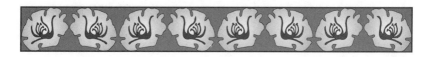

empire." Accepting Clarity as a value, we keep our bodies and environment clean; we try to reduce the amount of garbage we produce and recycle what we can; we care for the beauty of our world and delight in creating beautiful, simple spaces in which to live our lives.

Just as dirt and clutter can destroy the serenity of our homes, selfishness, pride, jealousy and rage can destroy the serenity of our minds. Embracing Shaoca means we commit ourselves to healing and thus "cleaning house". We begin to see our ego's defenses for what they are: clever devices to keep us in hell, when heaven is just a thought away. Marianne Williamson describes the "hell" many of our generation live through daily:

...Our oppression is internal. The government isn't holding us back, or hunger or poverty. We're not afraid we'll get sent to Siberia. We're just afraid, period. Our fear is free-floating. We're afraid this isn't the right relationship or we're afraid it is. We're afraid they won't like us or we're afraid they will. We're afraid of failure or we're afraid of success. We're afraid of dying young or we're afraid of growing old. We're more afraid of life than we are of death.

Fear is a deadly mental virus that can rage out of control when we live our lives in reaction to our world. Cleaning up our minds involves honestly facing our fears, naming them, and committing ourselves to their healing. If our fear wears the face of greed, we can practice consciously doing one unselfish act each day. If it wears the mask of anger, we can practice one act of kindness. P.R. Sarkar says that the simple, conscious act of being polite can heal someone afflicted with a pattern of anger or egoism. He says "Those who are very angry or egoistic ought to practice the h[...] of being polite; they serve humanity through that pra[...] Therefore, selfless service to humanity and the effort to lo[...] the world with a cosmic outlook alone can lead a pe[...] established in mental Shaoca."

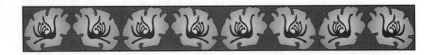

Shaoca in Our Relationships

Having clean, clear relationships takes work. It requires being honest all the time and having the courage to talk about what is in our hearts. When we live our lives trying to avoid pain, we take the crooked path. We don't realize that honesty is food for our spirits, and that our spirits begin to die of starvation when we begin to lie, to hide our true selves, to cover our feelings with a mask of invulnerability. Sometimes we need to move in the direction of pain in order to release it and find joy.

In 1989 I fell from a twelve-foot loft and tore the ligaments in my shoulder. I had constant pain for two years, and finally the shoulder "froze"—it literally stopped working and began to be excruciatingly painful all the time. Everything I had to do to heal it made the pain worse. Going to physical therapy three times a week for six months was like entering a torture chamber. I had to have it "unstuck" surgically at one point, and the subsequent therapy to keep it that way was even worse than before. Each time I faced the decision of whether to move further into the pain or not, it was a difficult choice. I knew if I didn't do something about it I would be in constant pain for an indefinite period of time, and would have to somehow live without the use of my arm. But it was unclear just how much progress I could make with physical therapy and surgery; there were no guarantees. I kept bringing up my courage and going forward, into more and ~~in, because I knew I had to do my part; I had to do every-~~l myself. Trying to avoid and minimize the

didn't want to be.

elationships as well. When we start
nflicts, we get stuck in a very small,
keep our feelings in, we must keep
s and our relationships clean requires
nto pain sometimes, in order to stay
v love in. A commitment to honesty

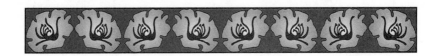

keeps the heartwaves clear.

With our children, Shaoca is more than bathing them every day and making them clean their rooms. If you watch children play in areas with and without fences, you will see that in a fenced playground they freely play in all the available space. They pop into the world of their imagination and explore. But without a fence, they clump together and fight, restricting the area they play in and avoiding the perimeters.

Children need the clarity of boundaries. The rules we set in our homes are like the fence; within these boundaries, they are secure and free to extend themselves. With no boundaries, they cannot explore; their spontaneity is limited and they either become fearful and withdrawn or reckless and aggressive. They will begin to act out in a subconscious effort to find the missing boundary line.

When boundaries do not exist, or when rules are arbitrary and enforced with rigidity, criticism and shame, children grow up with boundary problems and find it difficult to know how to act appropriately. For example, someone who has boundary problems doesn't expect to have to pick up his own clothes at home; borrows things and doesn't return them; ridicules, bullies or abuses his or her spouse, children or friends; presumes upon others by entering their homes, taking things, extending a loan, etc. without their permission. People who have grown up without clear boundaries find it difficult to say "yes" to healthy relationships and "no" to unhealthy ones; they find themselves in roles of victim and victimizer, carrying around a lot of shame and rage from all their failed relationships.

For peace in our homes, we need clear boundaries which include negotiable and non-negotiable rules. The non-negotiable rules should be reasonable and few. For example: (I use the words "may" and "may not" because these are the words I used with my own kids to indicate a non-negotiable rule)

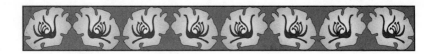

Toddler: You may not pull the cat's tail.
Young child: You may not cross the street without an adult.
Older child: You may not watch television on school nights.
Teenager: You may not drive my car without my permission.

Negotiable rules are those which can be discussed and some-what modified, with parents and children coming to an agreement on a case-by-case basis. For example:

Toddler: When we go to the store, you can choose a treat from the selections I provide.
Young child: On weekends and vacation days you can help decide your bedtime.
Older child: You can use the sewing machine with my help on Saturday morning.
Teenager: You can go out on a date, but I must know where you are and when I can expect you to be home.

Rules help children see where the "fence" that protects them starts and ends. There are both natural and logical consequences to all behavior. Logical consequences are those that are imposed when the natural consequences would be too dangerous or inappropriate. For example, the natural consequence of a toddler pulling the cat's tail would be getting scratched. But this is not a good risk for parents to allow. So a logical consequence needs to be clearly given by the parent. Logical consequences are best given in two or three stages. In this case, the parent could say, "No," physically remove the child's hand from the cat's tail and show the child how to pet the cat gently, saying, "Kitties are for petting. Pet the kitty gently," smiling and rewarding gentle petting with strokes and kisses. If the behavior continued after a few of these efforts, the parent would move on to the next stage,

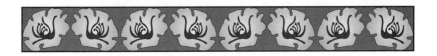

saying, "No. Kitties are for petting, not for hurting," and remove the child from the cat. The third stage (depending on the age-appropriateness for the child) could be a "time out" sitting on a chair. Rules require both clear (but non-abusive), negative consequences for breaking the rule and positive consequences for succeeding.

While parents sometimes need to let their children know about feelings connected with their actions ("I feel frustrated and angry when I find that you have been watching television after school"), consequences should be given with clarity and without excessive emotion: "You may watch television only on weekends. This rule is made for the peace of our household and so that you can grow up healthy. It is not negotiable. Watching television after school breaks the rule. The first time you break this rule, you will not be able to watch television the following weekend. The second time, the television will be unplugged and put away in the basement for two weeks. The third time, you will be grounded. My trust in you will be shaken." The most important part of this clarity of boundaries is that parents calmly and consistently follow up, and be willing to sacrifice their own time and energy to do so. When children know their boundaries, they rarely test them past the first or second violation.

Sometimes we need to look at our own behavior and how our children may be mirroring it. If we cannot follow through, communicate clearly, do our share and make amends for our mistakes, the natural consequences may be children who ignore the rules and are sullen, insolent, tardy, disrespectful, and who distrust us. We can begin to notice when we are communicating with rigidity, criticism, hypocrisy, passivity or abandonment, and try to think of ways we can move into clarity. We need to help our children trust us by following our own rules and following up clearly when they are broken.

Giving structure to our children's lives is one of the trials and

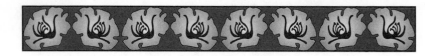

gifts of parenthood. The more clean and clear we are able to be in all our communications, the more our homes will be safe places of serenity for our kids.

Shaoca in Our Social and Political Choices

Embracing the ethic of Shaoca, we become aware of how we interact with our environment and what impact our personal choices have on it. Politically, we can get involved in alternative solutions to local ecological problems and we can use the power of constituency to influence those who make the nation's policies. We can ask ourselves:

1. *How much garbage do I produce each day?* What does it consist of? How can I reduce it? What measures has my community, my state, my country taken to address this issue? By using our food scraps for garden compost, recycling paper, plastic, glass, aluminum and whatever else we can, we contribute a great deal to the future health and cleanliness of our communities.

2. *How much water do I use, and how much do I waste?* Where does my water come from? How clean is it? What steps can I take to conserve water and ensure it will be clean and available in the future? Many futurists warn that a global water crisis is inevitable if we do not begin to pay attention to how we use and misuse this precious gift of life.

3. *How much of what I own serves a valuable purpose in my life?* How much is unnecessary and not of use to me? A good way to clean up our homes is to recycle the clothing, tools, kitchen items, toys, and other "stuff" we no longer use by donating them to charities which can repair, give or resell them to others.

4. *How clean is the air I breathe?* What steps can I take to reduce air pollution, both inside and outside my home?

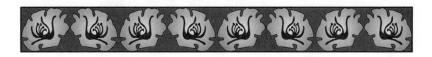

5. *Are there environmental hazards in my region?* How can I effect change and help protect my area from these hazards?

6. *Is there beauty and simplicity in my life?* How do I feel in the atmosphere and physical setting of my home, my vehicle, my property, my workplace? Does it enhance my mental peace? What steps can I take to change my environment so that it does so? Can I introduce artwork or other objects to beautify it? Would plants or animals like to share my space and add to its wholeness and balance? (And can I commit to serving them?) Can I change the color or lighting or introduce soothing fragrances? Can I reduce clutter and thus increase clarity? Is there a special place I can go to meditate and nourish my spirit?

Affirmation of Shaoca
Today I choose to be clean and clear in thought, word and action. I behave with clarity in all my relationships. I contribute to the beauty of my world.

Observe, Reduce, & Heal:	Practice:
Being disorganized	Paying attention to my surroundings as a reflection of my inner being
Staying stuck in crisis	Learning to accept events as neutral and accept my power and responsibility for changing what is not healthy
Irresponsible behavior toward my environment and possessions	Taking steps toward cleaning up my surroundings, my environment, my world
Habitual destructive expressions of emotion	Habitual supportive, loving expressions of emotion

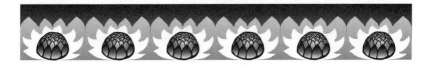

Chapter Seven
SANTOSA (sun-*toh*-shuh): Acceptance

"Acceptance is the magic that makes change possible."
—Melody Beattie

"Tosa" means a state of mental ease. Santosa is the contentment that comes from accepting ourselves and others just the way
we are. It is not the passive denial of our power; it is not a
surrender to fear. Rather, Santosa is the practice of choosing love
over fear in our everyday lives. Fear and all its accompanying reactions goads us into frantic activity or drags us into frozen depres-
sion. When we realize we have a choice, and when we make that
choice toward love, our lives come into balance and we begin to
feel contented.

Santosa in Our Personal Lives

The joy that is the result of practicing acceptance can only be
ours when we begin with ourselves. If we do not accept ourselves
at this moment, we cannot access love in our relationships or for
the betterment of our world. Self acceptance is not an easy practice in a dysfunctional society. The mirrors we face every day—on
television, in magazines, at work, in the marketplace—stare back
at us with disapproval. We can never be thin enough, rich
enough, smart enough, successful enough, or even happy enough!
When we react to this pressure from our own unhealed pain, we
feel driven, desperate, and unhappy. Happiness is just out of
reach; perfection is just around the corner. Serenity is out of the
question.

To practice Santosa we must begin to look honestly at our lives
and what drives us. I was driven for much of my early adult life
by experiences I had in childhood and adolescence which I had

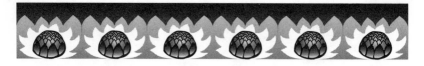

completely blocked out of my memory. I had decided to "be a new person," to start over with a new life when I left home to marry at 18. But I would get into patterns of fear and reaction, withdrawal and isolation, over and over again, not realizing that I had any choices. I was terrified of change, I worked in a frenzy, I simmered with resentment about my "fate" and I often felt isolated, lonely and defeated. It wasn't until I began to face those memories—to go back to those times and connect them with myself again—that I could begin to accept who I am and make empowering choices. Whatever we avoid in life ends up controlling us.

When we embrace and accept ourselves—our "dark" side with its rage, its shame, its fears and insecurities, its need to hide and control, as well as our "light" side and all our positive qualities—we can begin to walk the path of human being. We can begin to define ourselves instead of allowing others to define us. We can make the choices which empower us and allow us to release patterns of reaction and behavior that do not work for us anymore.

I was finally able to begin healing the pain which caused me to live in fear, and to learn new ways of thinking and behaving that helped me feel contented and return to center when my fears were triggered. I learned to accept myself and others, to express my feelings, to cultivate supportive relationships. I learned to accept change, to reduce stress, and to set limits for myself. I learned to express anger appropriately and to explore the feelings underlying my anger. I learned to take care of myself, to be loyal to myself, and to tell the truth about how I think and feel. I learned to live through uncomfortable times, to wait for clarity, to let go of the past and live in the here-and-now. And I learned to trust that my higher power is always with me. All of this is a part of the Santosa I now try to practice each day.

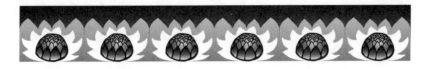

Santosa in Our Relationships

Practicing Santosa in our relationships requires that we accept the things we cannot change, to change the things we can, and to learn the difference. A relationship is always changing because we are always changing. Our relationships have the power to teach us the most important lessons we came here to learn, and so the more intimate and committed a relationship is, the more it teaches us. Even passing acquaintances can help us practice acceptance and thus allow the light of peace to shine from our eyes. An encounter with a sales clerk or a police officer or the mail carrier mirrors our consciousness and gives us another chance to bring love and healing to the world.

A primary relationship is the most powerful teacher we have, whether we actually have a primary relationship or not! If we are in a committed relationship, there is a struggle as our partner stimulates all the hidden craziness in us. If we are not in a committed relationship, there is still a struggle. Often the absence of a partner in itself makes us crazy and forces us to deal with our hidden pain.

Acceptance is a powerful attitude. We can accept a situation and yet choose to change it. We can accept others and still have choices. The ego sometimes fools us into mixing up acceptance and denial. A woman who "accepts" the abusive behavior of a violent spouse has not accepted him; rather, she is denying the truth. When she truly accepts the fact of the abuse, she can choose to get out and get help. A man who "accepts" that he has a violent temper and goes on abusing his spouse or children has not accepted himself; rather, he is denying the truth. When he truly accepts the fact of the abuse, he can choose to get out and get help.

Convincing ourselves that we have no choice is a sly defense against accepting our power. It keeps fear in control of our lives and keeps love and intimacy as far away as possible. Why do we

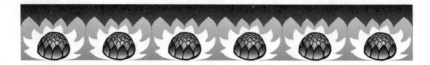

want to keep love away? Because true love shines a light on us and requires us to look at and heal a mountain of pain. Until we are ready to do that, the dull pain of unconscious fear is a familiar refuge—much preferable to the sharp pain of discovering and accepting things about ourselves we'd rather not look at, and the unknown realm of learning new ways of being. As long as we can blame others for our pain we can avoid the work of changing and its accompanying anxiety.

Practicing Santosa in our intimate relationships helps us learn to influence rather than control. We learn not to load others' behavior with so much "charge"; to negotiate and compromise to get our needs met and to help our partners meet their needs. We learn to ask ourselves, "How important is this?" We learn to roll with life; to accept others' foibles, failings, idiosyncracies and fears. Life is no longer a crisis because we choose contentment.

Practicing Santosa with our children helps them grow up feeling secure and loved, with lots of healthy personal power and self-esteem. Young children need to be cared for, to be touched and told they matter. They need to be noticed and accepted exactly as they are. Sometimes parents, under the influence of our own woundedness, think that our job is to straighten our kids out. So every communication, every instance of eye contact, is charged with shame, humiliation, disapproval, correction, and criticism. This is all well-intentioned; most parents want to do the right thing and are fearful of going wrong in such a way that our children don't "turn out right." What we don't realize is that belittling, pushing, criticizing or neglecting behavior is deeply harmful to our children and has the effect of making them into exactly what we fear. Santosa is unconditional love. It says, "I love you because you are here. I am glad you are my child. You deserve love; no strings attached." Both abuse and neglect interfere with a child's development and perpetuate the chain of pain. The wounded child is a wounded adult, who hurts himself and

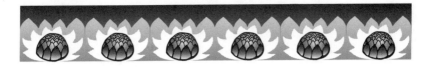

others and contributes to the making of a cold and violent society.

If you think your child is unaccepting of himself or herself, is converting your loving messages to criticism, or is feeling ashamed, investigate. Is there someone in the child's life who is interfering with his or her healthy development? Has your child been abused by someone, now or in the past? If this is true, you must get help and you must protect your child. If you suspect your own parenting responses have been inconsistent or detrimental, talk to your child about it, and make a conscious commitment to change and to help your child accept your love.

For example, if you feel your child didn't accept a loving message, tell him you aren't sure he heard you, and ask him to listen as you say it again. Tell her you're not sure she received what you said in the way you meant it, and would like a chance to say it again another way. (Don't expect a response; it takes time for children to learn to feel safe enough to respond). Say it to yourself. Does it sound loving to you? If not, re-word it until it does. Look for models in your life you can "copy" to learn loving, responsive behaviors.

Ask your child what he or she needs to hear; you'd be surprised at how clear they can be about what they want and need. If the child can't say, it is probably because he or she is frozen with fear around feeling and expressing. Try to create an atmosphere of safety, acceptance and support in which negative feelings can be expressed without punishment. Teach your children how to express their negative feelings in a way that doesn't cause harm to themselves or their relationships. Above all, listen to your children with respect and an open heart. Santosa provides an atmosphere in which a child can be fully human, test his boundaries safely, and grow up accepting himself and others. It creates a world which is loving and responsive, in which we all can thrive.

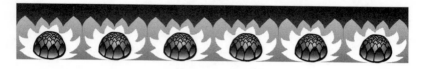

Santosa in Our Social and Political Choices

Santosa enables us to find a perspective when we are dealing with social and political injustice. Some social activists reject spirituality because they fear that it might engender a passive acceptance of exploitation; indeed, religious dogma has given rise to such passivity and to its opposite—rigidity which leads to war. But true spirituality and a practice of Santosa are not rigid or passive. P.R. Sarkar, in *A Guide to Human Conduct* says:

> Santosa Sadhana [practice] does not imply that someone should exploit you or oppress you by taking advantage of your simplicity and you should tolerate it silently. It is by no means proper to give up your right for self-preservation or your legitimate dues. You will have to go on fighting with joint efforts for the establishment of your rightful claim. But never go against the principle of Santosa, wasting your physical and mental energy under the sway of excessive greed.

Practicing Santosa, we allow ourselves to face reality and accept what is. We fight injustice not out of fear, anger and revenge, but with a love that gives us courage. When Christ admonished his followers to "turn the other cheek" I believe he meant that we must work to stay centered when we are threatened with aggression, oppression and exploitation. When we do not allow ourselves to get sucked into the fear that such a situation generates, we can act with courage and resolve to protect ourselves, our loved ones, and the earth from those whose pain has caused them to act out the ego's fearful dreams. Without the awareness of Santosa, we are easily pulled into the same negative energy we are fighting against.

I remember in the anti-war movement (during the war in Viet Nam) there were rings made out of the remains of American planes shot down over North Viet Nam. These were coveted by some of the elite of the movement; a sort of status symbol. The ideological principle was that of "swords into plowshares", but

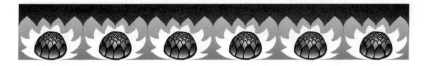

many of us couldn't help thinking of the families of the men who were in those planes; the grief and pain they were experiencing made the symbol and its message hollow and unreal.

Santosa is the practice of making ourselves quiet so as not to be at the mercy of our anger, our outrage, our feelings of injustice. In *How Can I Help?* Ram Dass and Paul Gorman talk about this "quiet mind."

> It takes the split-second timing of the quiet mind, working in harmony with the open heart, to know just when and how to say, "Hey!" to a potentially dangerous opponent. So we work to be clear enough to seize the time. If you're a union leader in a tough collective bargaining session, for example, you'll want to catch that moment when it's best to yield a little, or when to shake your head, 'No deal.' If you're working in a peace movement, timing will be crucial: when to call a national action, when to concentrate on local efforts; when to work on legislative opinion; when to confront the central government. With so much at stake, we need to strengthen that spacious awareness which allows us to take in all the elements of a political situation.

In recent years and throughout history, seemingly invulnerable institutions and political systems have crumbled into nothing overnight. Practicing Santosa helps us see through the frightening masks of oppression and injustice and work consistently for unity and peace. In *The Wizard of Oz*, Dorothy found that the boastful lion masked a frightened child; the all-powerful wizard was only a fearful little man trying to get his needs met. As long as she remained a slave to her fear, she was powerless; an act of loving courage allowed the mask to fall away and the truth to be revealed. The terrifying witch evaporated when the forces of good found their center and acted with courage and unity. Finally, Dorothy discovered that she had the power to return home all along—it was all in her mind. All of the world's myths and legends focus on these themes: that courage is required to slay the dragons, to defeat the evil empire, to overcome the devil and the

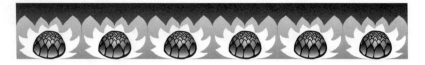

forces of darkness; that love always triumphs over the illusory spectre of hatred; and that outward change can happen only when we change our own minds.

When we live every day with the act of faith in a higher power, when we choose not to succumb to fear, every circumstance in which we find ourselves enriches and strengthens us. When bad things happen, it is those whose love is strong and clear, who are capable of accepting truth and acting with faith, on whom others rely. There was a deeply touching film (*The Hiding Place*)—a true story—about some Christian women who, as a result of their efforts to protect and defend hundreds of Dutch Jews from the Nazis, were captured and sent to a concentration camp. One of these women in particular was able somehow to keep her faith in God alive through the horrors going on all around her. She continued to work to help others, not in an aggressive or bold manner, but quietly, with calm acceptance. She risked her life every day to help others who were not able to find faith or courage or hope. At one point she said, "There is no darkness that is so deep that I will not find God when I go deeper still." This resolve, this firmly and quietly chosen belief, is what the practice of Santosa is all about.

Affirmation of Santosa

Today I choose to be contented. I accept myself and I accept others as they are. I accept the world as it is, and choose to contribute to its healing.

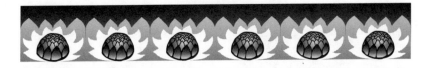

Observe, Reduce, & Heal:	Practice:
An addiction to struggle & crisis	Recognizing past patterns; willingness to feel contentment
A habit of being a victim	Being loyal to myself; clarifying my choices; choosing to own my power to heal myself
Dependence on others for self-definition	Accepting myself and choosing my own ways of being
Chronic unhappiness & addiction to more & more material solutions	Meditation, contemplation, helping and serving others; focusing on the non-material benefits of life
Negative focus on the past or future	Willingness to live in the present
Jealousy of others' accomplishments, personalities, material wealth	Acts of kindness and generosity

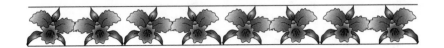

Chapter Eight
TAPAH (*tah*-pah): Sacrifice

"We must alter our lives in order to alter our hearts, for it is impossible to live one way and pray another."

—Saint Paul

Tapah has undergone several incarnations in its definition. In Patanjali's time, Tapah implied the mortification of the body to reach higher states of consciousness. Yoga practitioners would sit in freezing water or in painful postures or would fast in an effort to rid themselves of the attachments of the physical body; many Christian monks and nuns did likewise. This is where the image of a yogi on a bed of nails came from. But later interpretations rejected these practices because they merely replace the attachment to pleasure with the attachment to pain, creating an unnatural aversion to everything that makes us human.

With later interpretations of Patanjali's work, Tapah came to be seen in a more positive light, meaning "self-discipline" or "self-restraint"—the attainment of a kind of self-sufficiency which allowed the yoga practitioner to release his attachments and thus rid himself of greed. But too much self-sufficiency is a kind of greed in itself. We are all part of a universe which requires our participation, our interdependence with other beings.

P.R. Sarkar defines Tapah (the real definition of which, after all, is "penance" or "sacrifice") as the conscious practice of giving of ourselves—sacrificing some of our time, energy, and material wealth— to help those who need help. He says:

A sick person is feeling uneasy owing to great pain; if you serve him for hours running to give him needed relief, this is Tapah; but if you serve him

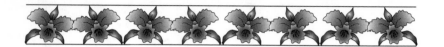

with a selfish motive to have a return in your bad days, the entire effort of Tapah is lost in a moment. Tapah sadhana [practice] is, therefore, to be above selfishness. ...There must be one and only one purpose behind this acceptance of penance and this is to shoulder sorrows and miseries to keep [those you serve] happy, to free them from grief and to give them comfort.

Practicing Tapah keeps us aware of our connection with others. In American society the word "sacrifice" implies a kind of sickness. We detest self-righteousness and the martyrdom of people who are enslaved to taking care of everyone but themselves. However, in healing ourselves of the compulsive other-centeredness of codependency, we sometimes throw out the baby with the bathwater, becoming more and more self-centered as we replace an obsession with pleasing others with obsessively taking care of ourselves.

Middle class life offers very little opportunity for children to learn the joy and the pain of serving their less fortunate brothers and sisters. In many third world cultures the children participate in the struggles of daily life. Their observation of their parents' sacrifices for others imbues in them a sense of human obligation to help, and with it, a trust in the natural order of things. American culture has little or no opportunity or support for this type of participation and learning. Suffering, deprivation and pain are sanitized and removed from our experience so that we view those who suffer with aversion and a pity which keeps us distant. With no daily relationship to suffering, the fear of it grows large and we work frenetically to keep "the wolf from the door." Because we have created a society in which we can live our entire lives not knowing our neighbors we have won freedom from social bonds—we have gained the privacy of individuality. But the price we have paid is dear. Defending ourselves against the suffering of others, we have invited another kind of suffering—that of loneliness, isolation and despair. And we have

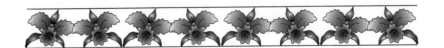

not gained security or safety in our isolation; suffering will come to us no matter how many walls we build around ourselves. If the pain of those who suffer from injustice doesn't come to burn down our homes or businesses, most of us will still have to face old age and illness without the security of a community which respects and cares for us. This is the nature of fear-based living; the very walls our egos build for protection become the prisons in which our spirits languish.

In *How Can I Help?* Ram Dass and Paul Gorman explore the ways in which we distance ourselves from others' pain and thus deprive our spirits of the opportunity to expand.

Denial, abstraction, pity, professional warmth, compulsive hyperactivity: these are a few of the ways in which the mind reacts to suffering and attempts to restrict or direct the natural compassion of the heart. This tension between head and heart leaves us tentative and confused. As we reach out, then pull back, love and fear are pitted against one another. As hard as this is for us, what must it be like for those who need our help?

...So we have to find tranquility in the midst of trauma. What's required is to cultivate a dispassionate Witness within. This Witness, as it grows stronger, can see precisely how we jump the gun in the presence of pain. It notices how our reactions might be perpetuating denial or fear or tension in the situation, the very qualities we'd like to help alleviate. The Witness catches us in the act, but gently, without reproach, so we can simply acknowledge our reactivity and begin to let it fall away, allowing our natural compassion to come more into play.

...Now we can begin, perhaps for the first time, to hear them. Less busy pushing away suffering, less frenzied having to do something about it, we're able to get a sense of what they're feeling, of what they feel they need.

Becoming overwhelmed by guilt or pity in the presence of suffering is a way for our ego/mind to get out of the heart and away from the opportunity to serve. For service, truly rendered, opens the heart and brings us into a simple, honest human place in which we realize our vulnerability and connection with others.

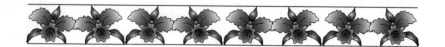

No way! says the ego, intent on maintaining the illusion of separation. I remember someone once telling me (after I had shared with her the joy of being in Mother Teresa's baby hospital in Calcutta), "I am just too sensitive for that. I just couldn't handle being in a place like India with all that suffering all around, and not being able to do anything about it! Why, it would be just too painful for someone like me. I guess that's why I was born in the United States."

Tapah in Our Personal Lives

Practicing Tapah—giving of ourselves to serve those in need— is one of the most powerful spiritual practices available to us. It awakens our hearts to our connection with others; it mirrors our unhealed places and gives us the opportunity to grow; and it gives us the chance to feel the support, the love—the energy—of our higher power in our lives.

Tapah is the act, however small, of quietly giving beyond what normally and naturally comes to us. It is not the routine writing of checks to foundations for the poor; nor is it the grandiose gesture which gets our name in the newspaper. It is neither other-centered nor self-centered. The secret of real Tapah is that it is done without any fanfare, it is done through sacrifice, and it is done simply for the sake of doing it.

Practicing Tapah, we become more available to whoever we are with; compassion and a sense of unity become increasingly automatic responses in all of our interactions. As we learn to nurture others, we experience being nurtured by a love that is greater than anything we've ever known.

This is the essence of the spiritual path of devotional service. One enters into the helping act not only because there is a need to be met. Service gradually becomes an offering, first to those we are with, but eventually to that greater truth or source of being in which we are all joined in love. Helping

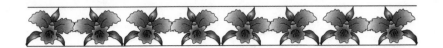

becomes an act of reverence, worship, gratitude. It is grace merely to have the chance to serve.

Mother Teresa, for example, bending to hold a dying leper, sees there only "Christ in a distressing disguise." She's not "helping a dying leper," she's loving God, affirming in whomever she's with universal qualities of perfection and beauty. One can imagine how it might feel to be held in this spirit during one's final moments of life.

—from *How Can I Help?* by Ram Dass and Paul Gorman

Practicing Tapah does not require us to go to Calcutta to work with Mother Teresa. We can find plenty of opportunities to practice right in our own backyards. We don't practice Tapah because we feel it is an important thing to do or that we are making a big difference. It is done simply because it is a part of being on this Earth. Some of the ways Americans have found to practice Tapah include:

• Making a commitment to help someone we know who is ill or injured.
• Participating in "meals-on-wheels" projects in which we have a chance to connect person-to-person with the people to whom we are taking food.
• Volunteering at a shelter for the homeless, for battered women, for abused and abandoned children, for people with AIDS, at a hospice for the dying.
• Volunteering to help with a local food distribution center or starting one ourselves.
• Being a foster parent or a "big brother" or sister.
• Teaching others to read through a literacy program.
• Volunteering on a hot-line service for suicide prevention or child abuse.
• Getting paramedical skills and volunteering in an ambulance, fire, or disaster service.

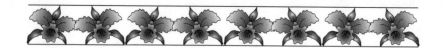

Tapah can include donating food, clothing or money to causes which help those in need, but real Tapah requires us to face those we serve and interact with them. It is sometimes very difficult to find time to serve others in this way; with family and career responsibilities, there are only so many hours in a day. For some, taking time off to do service works better; we may volunteer for a year in the Peace Corps or take vacation time to work in a service project full time. When we are open to them, opportunities to grow through sacrifice come to us; we don't need to look very far.

Tapah in Our Relationships
Every relationship requires Tapah in order to grow. Love cannot be given, cannot be experienced, without a sacrifice of the ego's attachment to selfishness and separation. Kimberly Heart, in her book *When Fairy Tale Romances Break Real Hearts* says the definition of fear is: F.E.A.R.—False Evidence Appearing Real. The ego produces fear in an effort to support faulty belief systems. For example, if in childhood we took in the belief that we are responsible for the happiness or pain of everyone around us, our ego's job is to uphold that belief and look for evidence to support it. Why? Because our ego's job is to maintain our individuality; our "me"-ness, our survival. So our egos have an important role. However, in a healthy person, the ego is subordinate to the soul or spirit, not the other way around. We get unhealthy when our spirits are crushed and our egos are given control of our lives. In this example, we find evidence to support this false belief; we read blame into others' pain. Aha! See? I *am* responsible for your pain! The ego then goes to work trying to fix the other person, solve the problem, etc. In the meantime, someone close to us is in pain and needs our emotional and spiritual support and connection—areas in which the ego flounders. We are so busy gathering False Evidence we cannot be in our hearts, and we end up causing further pain rather than fixing, solving or healing anything. This

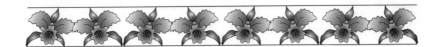

false evidence can appear so real to us that we completely miss the real cries for help that may be coming our way.

When I fell and badly injured my arm, my husband and I went through a kind of crisis in our relationship. I was in constant pain, taking heavy drugs and completely unable to do anything for myself or anyone else. I was also in a constant state of terror; afraid of the pain, which was nearly unbearable; afraid of the physical therapy (which increased it); afraid I would be crippled for the rest of my life.

My husband had never taken care of someone who was sick or in pain, and had little experience with the emotional challenges an illness can cause. Like it or not, it was time for him to practice Tapah. It would have been difficult for anyone. Thinking about it now, I still don't know if I'd have changed places with him. I had some pretty big lessons myself, but his were no less challenging. I asked him to talk about it, and have transcribed what he said here:

What I learned from the whole ordeal we went through after my wife's injury was to put myself in her place. I had to start thinking more of her as if she were me. That's what marriage is supposed to be about— taking our partner's needs to be as important as our own.

At first when my wife's body was in terrible, frightening pain and she needed emotional support from me, I was busy problem solving. My ego had a fearful reaction to her pain; my mind kept asking, "Is this my fault? and… What can I do to make sure it's not my fault any more?" The harder I tried, the more upset and frustrated she became because what she needed was emotional support and an all-around nurturing presence from me. As I got into that problem-solving mode and she became more frustrated, I read her frustration as dissatisfaction with me and rejection of my efforts. My ego went crazy trying to convince me she was doing this out of spite and I should just shut down. I lost touch with my heart and got way into my mind. My heart became completely inaccessible to me, and that just confirmed my diagnosis that I was not a good person, and her diagnosis that I didn't really care about her.

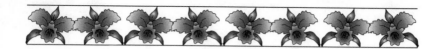

We kept going around in circles. Our love for each other would allow us to try to patch things up, but then her pain would get to a crisis point and the relationship would fall apart again. I would offer something and get no feedback from her. She would get angry at my lack of compassion. I would get angry at her seeming rejection of my perfectly good solutions. We would get polarized and separated.

It is amazing how our minds construct evidence of inadequacy which serves to distance us from the people we are trying to help. At first it never even occurred to me that receptivity was the key to being of help. It wasn't my ability, but my *availability* that was required. Making ourselves available means opening ourselves, making ourselves vulnerable to pain. The ego doesn't want that! So it jumps in, trying to get control of the situation.

I finally got to the point when I was so frustrated with this whole cycle I just let it go; I decided, okay—fine. I'm not a good person, I'm not a good caregiver. I'm just going to accept that and accept myself. I can't do anything about her reaction to me or her pain but I can do something with myself. I started trying to work on forgiveness with myself and accepting the whole situation the way it was. When I did that, I started getting back in touch with my heart, and I started getting more response from her. I needed to learn that it wasn't about me healing her, or taking charge and making it all better. It was about a quiet acceptance of what was going on; just being present; just listening.

I think when we're confronted with anybody's pain, fear is a reflex. We must simply accept everything about the situation, including our own emotions and reactions. Instead of going with the fear, the first step is just to work on accepting it all. When we go with the fear, we shut off our own ability to provide help. I thought I was scared of my inability to do the right things. But I found that I know intuitively what to do when I'm quieted down, in a listening space. It's built into us to know what to do.

My real fear was about the intimacy of sharing someone's pain. And that's all about the spirit versus the ego being in charge of our lives. True spirituality brings true intimacy, which is a kind of sacrifice. It's laying ourselves on the altar in surrender. Our egos construct evidence of a vengeful universe that will cut us open. But what actually happens is we are touched with a feather and blessed. True service is about getting on that altar and laying ourselves bare in spite of what our egos are telling us might happen.

This experience helped me realize that the most profound gift we can give those who suffer in our presence is peace. To stop the shouting of our egos, the searching for validation. It's like we have two buttons, send and receive. Service

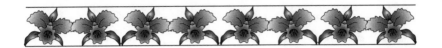

is about turning off the send button and switching to receive. To quiet down and become an empty vessel, available to receive anything.

Tapah, then, is a personal sacrifice; the surrender of the ego. In a relationship, Tapah is what increases the level of intimacy between partners or friends. People who never extend themselves to help one another—who never allow vulnerability or service into their relationship—limit its depth and commitment. Intimate relationships are practice for our relationship with our deepest selves; our relationship with God.

Children are the best teachers of Tapah we can possibly have. In order to be good parents we must be willing to sacrifice for our kids; to stretch ourselves beyond our fear and limitations. Walking the baby all night long, changing diapers, developing routines in which our children can feel safe and protected, planning for their education, providing medical care, emotional support, boundaries and freedom—all require us to give of ourselves, to re-organize our lives and our priorities. Parenting goes wrong when the spirit of Tapah is lost and fear takes over.

One of the important reasons teenage pregnancy is often a tragedy is that two very powerful forces of growth are required at the same time, and this double-bind is nearly impossible to negotiate. The teenage years are a time of individuation, when the ego goes into full swing because of the fear generated by separation from parents and home. It is thus a time when we are selfish and self-centered; we have a difficult time understanding others and giving of ourselves for their welfare. When individuation has been achieved and our fears are assuaged, we're ready to put our spirits back in the driver's seat and to grow through sacrifice.

The core requirement of good parenting is the ability to place a child's needs ahead of our wants; to feel safe and centered ourselves so that we can provide safety and balance to our children. How can a teenager possibly achieve both of these phases of

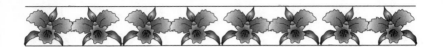

growth at the same time? It's no wonder that children of teenaged parents are often abused and neglected.

Tapah in Our Social and Political Choices

Tapah is often called "selflessness" but this term has a negative connotation in Western society. It is not so much about being selfless as it is about practicing the release of our fears—*egolessness.* It is not about losing ourselves in others, or neglecting our own needs, our mental peace, or our health to be there for other people. Occasionally, this "emergency" mode of service is required; an accident or a disaster may require temporary service from us in which we completely put aside our normal lives and our everyday needs. However, if we find ourselves in a lifestyle of emergency and crisis, something is wrong. We can practice sacrifice as a part of our everyday lives, just as we practice clarity or acceptance.

If we feel that Tapah is more important than Santosa (contentment; acceptance) so that we lose our balance and succumb to "burnout", there is pain inside us that needs healing. Carmen Renee Berry talks about this in her book *When Helping You is Hurting Me.* She describes the unhealthy side of service as "The Messiah Trap," saying that in order to avoid dealing with suppressed pain, we often become "helpaholics." We begin to try to live by a contradictory belief system that asserts 1) If I don't do it, it won't get done, and 2) Everyone else's needs take priority over mine. The first makes us feel superior to others and powerful; the second makes us feel worthless and powerless. So we're always one-up or one-down to others; it becomes impossible to just be a human being with everybody else. She says:

> These Messiahs neglect themselves because they feel that they are supposed to sacrifice their own well-being for the sake of others. This is the Messiah definition of love. Messiahs view life as a series of choices—choices between their

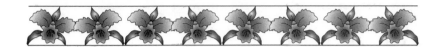

needs and the needs of others. It is as if the Messiah believes that there is only a limited amount of nurturance, caring, and love to go around—only enough for everyone else but nothing left over for the Messiah.

Consequently, there can grow inside of a Messiah a gnawing, hard-to-describe feeling. Sometimes it feels like being underappreciated for sacrifices made. Other times it feels more like guilt when taking time for personal needs somehow means having to disappoint or neglect someone else. Many times the feeling is fatigue, a deep tiredness that seems too heavy to carry. Most often Messiahs are too busy to feel anything at all except for the pressure of having too much to do and too little time. When Messiahs feel overwhelmed and underappreciated, most respond by helping even more.

Politically, we have come to value cleverness more than sincerity. The media portrays a sincere politician as stupid and encourages admiration of those who are smooth and can give seamless performances. We have come to take for granted that a politician must be selfish, greedy, and business-like. Politics is currently a business career, not one of service. We expect a politician to do things only because they serve his or her own career interests; if that happens to coincide with doing something good for society, great. Is something wrong here?

At some point we will begin to use human values as a measuring stick: How has this candidate demonstrated honesty in his or her professional and personal life? How congruent are his or her words and actions? And finally: Does this candidate have experience in service? Has he or she sacrificed for others less fortunate? Does he or she demonstrate an ethic of service when the cameras are not rolling?

Affirmation of Tapah

Today I open my heart to myself and others. I am willing to extend myself in service to someone in need. I trust my higher power to guide me.

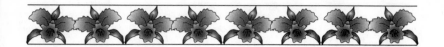

Observe, Reduce, & Heal:	Practice:
Making myself indispensable	Offering my service in cooperation with others
Rescuing and advising people	Taking care of myself; detaching from the need to rescue and advise
Ignoring my own needs	Setting limits for helping others
Losing my identity in others	Developing my own identity and interests
Self-centered lifestyle	Making time to help others less fortunate

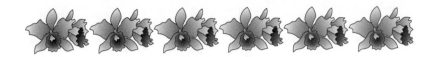

Chapter Nine
SVADHYAYA (swahd-*yah*-yah): Understanding

"We do not want churches. They will teach us to quarrel about God."
—Chief Joseph, in *Bury My Heart at Wounded Knee*

In ancient India, Svadhyaya was the study of spiritual scriptures. It implies the use of the mind to understand how the universe works. It is much more than reading books or listening to sermons; true understanding requires an effort to grasp the underlying significance of spiritual ideas—to use our rational judgment in concert with our feelings and intuition.

Svadhyaya in Our Personal Lives

Understanding, as a spiritual practice, is a commitment to the truth. We learn to listen and to read with our hearts, and to use our minds to filter out the garbage and find the gems. Every religion, every spiritual teaching has gems of true knowledge. But these are often cloaked in the dogma which armors the egos of so-called religious people driven by fear. Daily spiritual practice—and particularly deep meditation—sharpens our intuitive faculties and helps us see through this armor.

We can follow any spiritual path we choose; it is our understanding which will bring us enlightenment and peace, not the rote practice of one thing or another. We take ourselves into heaven or hell by choosing whether our hearts or our egos will run our lives. The mind is like the very best of tools. In the hands of an artist it can create beauty; in the hands of a homicidal maniac, it can destroy life. When the mind is used by the heart, with compassion, we grow in knowledge and understanding. When the mind is used by the ego, with fear and hatred, we grow

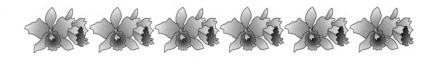

hard and our world contracts.

I have always thought of Svadhyaya as the practice of fine-tuning what I call my nonsense sensor. It's that radar-of-the-heart that tells me something's wrong. It tends to go off when I hear or read something that makes no sense; something which condemns, judges, or maligns; something which sounds like fear masquerading as spiritual or religious teaching. Meditation can sharpen this faculty if it is done wholeheartedly, with consciousness. Reading spiritual books can give us practice in understanding our own spirituality and broadening our perspective. Svadhyaya is the practice of looking deeper.

Svadhyaya in Our Relationships

In our relationships, Svadhyaya can have many implications. We can commit ourselves to discovering the underlying forces which cause the feelings we have or which cause us to behave the way we do. Intimacy thrives in an environment of exploration. I call it being soft to the truth. When we can soften and listen we make ourselves available to true understanding. How many times have we heard or said, "You just don't understand!"? What we're saying is, "I don't feel heard." When we are truly heard there is a sense of relief in our hearts. The fear drains away and we become available to ourselves and others again. But it is sometimes so hard to listen without fear!

I worked with parents and infants for twelve years, teaching massage techniques as a way to strengthen relationships. Through this daily contact with parents and infants I discovered that the one and only problem infants have is not being heard. Massage became the vehicle through which I could help parents learn how to listen to their babies. When an infant is finally listened to wholeheartedly, everything changes. Colic clears up, the baby relaxes and begins to really shine with his or her inherent joy. Most people don't realize that babies have as much to talk about

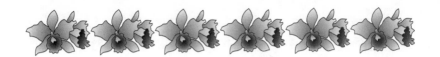

as we do; that they need to ventilate emotions and have their feelings received with love and acceptance. So do children. And so do adults. But often we respond by hardening our hearts, armoring for war. Someone else's pain can trigger fear and a reminder of the anguish and rage we may have felt as children, crying alone in a crib with no response; unable to express negative feelings and have them received. It can also engender guilt (am I a bad person if I caused this pain?) which often leads to anger and revenge as our egos try to defend against a perceived attack.

Learning how to listen with our hearts is one of the most valuable contributions we can make to our relationships—including our relationship with ourselves. A listening heart provides an atmosphere in which exploration of all the layers can take place.

Svadhyaya in our Social and Political Choices

In our social lives, Svadhyaya is that which brings us a deeper knowledge and understanding of social and political forces. The media reduces all our news to the lowest common denominator—to either-or and all-or-nothing choices—and so we find ourselves taking simplistic stands about issues on which we have little information. Svadhyaya is the refusal of the simplistic; the effort to get the information and make rational choices. It is the process of listening to what social leaders and politicians are saying between the lines, and applying human moral standards to our beliefs. Racism, sexism, ageism, injustice of any kind is a product of fear. When we react with fear rather than responding with love and understanding, war breaks out.

We all fear the hard realities of where our society is headed, because in our hearts we know that what goes out from us comes back to us. There are no longer any simple answers to our social problems; big, big changes will have to happen before we can begin to grow healthy again. Our economic system is destroying our environment, and saving our environment will require a total

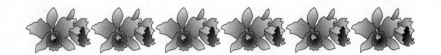

restructuring of our way of life. Providing a healthy environment for every human being, plant and animal must eventually become our one and only mission, for which we are willing to change the way we live right now. Practicing Svadhyaya—reading, listening, trying to understand the truth—can help us individually change in ways that support the healthy change of our communities and our world.

Affirmation of Svadhyaya

Today I seek a deeper understanding of life. I am willing to see things differently. I read and listen with an open mind and heart in order to form compassionate, responsible opinions.

Observe, Reduce, & Heal:	Practice:
Attachment to fear-based beliefs which are racist, sexist, ageist, or socially irresponsible	Choosing beliefs which are compassionate, accepting, and empowering for all life
Overreacting to change	Accepting change
Being judgmental and rigid	Accepting others as they are; reading and listening to discover common ground
Inability to listen to others' pain	Learning how to listen with my heart
Tendency to take advice or teachings at face value; to cling to the "letter of the law"	Trying to perceive and follow the "spirit of the law"
Voting or expressing opinions with no information (forexample,voting Republican or Democratic simply because I'm registered that way)	Reading and asking questions in order to vote and form responsible opinions

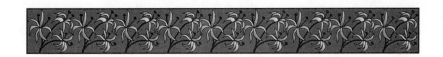

Chapter Ten
IISHVARA PRANIDHANA
(eesh-*war*-uh prah-nee-*dahn*):
Spirituality

"We're here to learn to go with joy among the sorrows of the world."
—Joseph Campbell

Iishvara Pranidhana is a mouthful; let's use the term spirituality. The literal meaning of Iishvara Pranidhana is "to take shelter in the Supreme"; this, to me, connotes a joyful surrender—a decision to make spirituality the point and purpose of our lives. Spirituality is both a value in itself and a result of choosing kindness, simplicity, honesty, acceptance, responsibility, unity, clarity, sacrifice and understanding in our everyday lives.

Spirituality can be expressed in many ways. In the yoga system, spirituality is both a practice and a sense, or feeling, about who we are which comes out of that practice. Time-tested techniques include yoga postures, which refine the body; healthy food, which calms and strengthens both body and mind; meditation, which refines the mind and nurtures the heart, and ethical behavior, which brings our hearts and minds together in relation to others and our world.

When spirituality is the core of our lives, it is as if a loving parent is watching over a growing child. It is said that the mind (and its outward expression, the ego) is a terrible master, but a wonderful servant. The only way to appropriately use the mind is to put our hearts in control of our physical, mental, emotional and spiritual well-being. In this context I equate the heart with what we may call soul or spirit; that aspect of our being which is

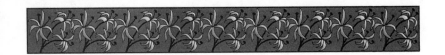

in harmony with unconditional love.

Setting aside time each day to pray or meditate in solitude helps us bring awareness to the rest of the day. Quieting the mind and directing its flow toward oneness with the inner Self allows us to re-experience the peace and joy which is the heart of all existence. Accessing this inner connection helps us to behave in ways which reflect our values, and thus our impact on the world around us is positive and profound.

American philosopher John Boodin said, "We are impelled by a hidden instinct to reunion with the parts of the larger heart of the universe." Whether we consciously acknowledge it or not, we move toward that reunion—that oneness—each time we choose to express love and release fear.

Joy

It is easy to see what is wrong. It takes practice to notice what is right. We must learn to identify and accept reality; but because we have been taught to see the world with fear, we often become habituated to equating reality with negativity. When we begin to see the world and our lives through the eyes of love we understand that joy is the fundamental reality of all existence, and that love can empower us even in the most painful times. Fear and hatred can be released. It is natural for us to feel pain sometimes, to experience "negative" emotions, to know the dark side of ourselves and our world. Denying this dark side keeps us from learning and growing. When we cannot feel intensely negative, we cannot feel intensely positive either; denial leads to frozen feelings and an inability to empathize with others. It is a kind of "positive negativity." But we can take the next step—into a positive, joyful way of seeing—and bring ourselves back into harmony. Negativity takes us out of harmony and gives power to our problems.

Choosing positive energy, we empower ourselves to find

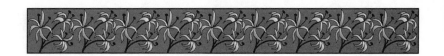

healthy solutions. Because we believe in love, we can face hatred. When we are no longer controlled by fear, we enter a new reality, where joy is an everyday feeling. We begin to notice all the beauty around us. Expressing and receiving love and support, we become accustomed to feeling safe and cared for. We move swiftly through sad feelings and problems as we become successful at negotiating life's terrain. Like expert sailors, we learn how to handle the storms and dangers; and we learn to love the sea. Pleasure, fun, enjoyment, laughter, intimacy, and spiritual joy—all become the reality of life for us.

To teach ourselves to live in joy, all we need to do is practice. Three exercises—performed each day like a musician playing scales—can help us find joy.

Count the Blessings

Consciously noticing all the good things empowers our lives with healthy positive energy. Each night before we go to sleep, we can take an inventory of all the good things that happened during the day. We can ask ourselves what is right, what is good—about our behavior and feelings, other people, our work, our relationships, our world. Wouldn't it be great if the evening news included at least equal time for *good* news? Since it doesn't, we can provide ourselves with good news each evening, and go to sleep feeling blessed. Says Melody Beattie, author of *The Language of Letting Go*:

Gratitude unlocks the fullness of life. It turns what we have into enough, and more. It turns denial into acceptance, chaos to order, confusion to clarity. It can turn a meal into a feast, a house into a home, a stranger into a friend. It turns problems into gifts, failures into successes, the unexpected into perfect timing, and mistakes into important events. It can turn an existence into a real life, and disconnected situations into important and beneficial lessons. Gratitude makes sense of our past, brings peace for today, and creates a vision for tomorrow.

Self-Analysis

Honesty makes room in our hearts for ourselves and each other. Once a week, we can take time to make a personal inventory of our lives and look bravely at our mistakes and behavior. An art teacher once said to me, "There is no such thing as a failure. Rather, we are successful at learning what we don't want to repeat."

Admitting we have behaved in a way we regret, or that we have made a mistake or unintentionally hurt someone helps us move into healing and joy. This can be threatening to our egos, which are fearful of being vulnerable. If we were shamed as children, feelings of shame may arise when we make mistakes. Instead of the healthy remorse out of which comes healing and change, we struggle with self-hatred. Shame breeds anger as the ego strives to protect us from the pain of self-annihilation. We put ourselves and others out of our hearts and the damage remains. Looking at our mistakes with kindness and courage, we become truly human. How often have we wished that someone who hurt or disappointed us could just acknowledge our pain and sincerely say, "I'm sorry"?

Regular self-analysis teaches us appropriate humility and makes room in our lives for growth. We can use Yama and Niyama as a guide for our inventory, discovering where we have unconsciously chosen fearful reactions when we could have chosen love. We can look for the ways in which our feelings, thoughts and behavior have reflected old patterns. We can also discover ways in which we have been successful at seeing the world with love. We can look for the ways in which our feelings, thoughts and behavior have reflected trust, faith, courage, self-esteem, honesty, unity, and understanding. Self-analysis is not to punish ourselves for wrong-doing; rather, it is a way to lovingly parent ourselves into wholeness.

Meditation

There are many ways to pray and meditate; each of us will discover, through study and exploration of various teachings, which practices stir our hearts and bring us forward. The most effective meditation practices cannot be given in a book; rather, an experienced and qualified teacher must be sought out. But there are some simple ways to begin, which can profoundly effect our outlook and behavior.

I have been practicing the Ananda Marga system of meditation for more than twenty years, and cannot recommend it highly enough. The meditation lessons are specific and, when carefully practiced, bring awareness, realization and rapid growth. The meditation itself unites heart and mind and brings us into an experience of a tremendous, universal love. It is then up to us, with the help of Yama and Niyama, to bring that flow into our daily behavior.

The Ananda Marga system includes a simple meditation on a *mantra*. The mantra is a Sanskrit phrase which brings the mind into harmony with universal love both because of its meaning and because of the impact of its intrinsic vibration upon the mind. The mantra used to prepare the mind for further lessons is *Baba Nam Kevalam* (pronounced *bah-bah nahm kay-vah-lum*) and is often sung before meditation to help bring our externally-focused energies into a spiritual flow. The meditator may then sit with eyes closed and repeat the mantra, allowing it to permeate and vibrate the mind and heart with its inner sound and meaning. *Baba Nam* means "the name of my beloved" and indicates the Supreme Consciousness, God, the Mother or whatever you may call the spiritual beloved of your life (words often fail us when we try to outwardly conceptualize the Supreme). *Kevalam* means "all-pervading." The meaning or ideation of the mantra is that God is love and every particle of the universe is God. We may find ways to phrase this which suit our taste; it is important that

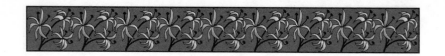

we meditate upon something which stirs our hearts and brings peace and unity to our minds. People have phrased the ideation in many ways: Love is all there is; the Infinite Consciousness is in everything; I am One with my Beloved; All is One.

Through the practice of spirituality in my own life, I have come to believe that spiritual progress is not limited to a specific doctrine or practice, though spiritual practices are essential to our growth. I believe that there are many systems of prayer and meditation which, when carefully, lovingly and sincerely practiced, bring about the unity of heart and mind which we seek.

One practice which I sometimes use to augment my own is in the Buddhist tradition. Stephen Levine teaches something like it, calling it "A Simple Loving Kindness Meditation" in his book, *Healing into Life and Death*. This "meditation" or blessing (a translation of a Sanskrit mantra or spiritually-empowered poem) is often given by great spiritual teachers at the close of their speeches. I believe it is a wonderful way to begin a daily meditation session, or to begin your spiritual journey while you are searching for the right teacher.

> Sit in a comfortable position in your special place, and close your eyes. Breathe deeply several times. Relax your body and mind and allow your attention to settle in the present. Allow your breath to come naturally as you release control and get into an open, receptive awareness. Begin to direct toward yourself the feeling of kindness. Feel as if you are breathing loving kindness into every cell. Observe your mind and how it relates or reacts to the words of the following blessing.
>
> Silently, slowly repeat: "May I dwell in the heart. May I be free from suffering. May I see the bright side of everything. May I be healed. May I be at peace." Continue repeating this blessing, allowing your body, mind and spirit to be filled with kindness and mercy.

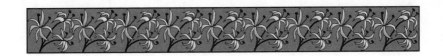

This blessing may be followed with meditation on a mantra, or following the breath, or whatever prayer or meditation practice you choose.

Imagine the world if everyone could say and feel this blessing every day, bringing all our thoughts, words, and actions into harmony with it.

Affirmation for Iishvara Pranidhana

May all beings dwell in the heart. May all beings be free from suffering. May all beings see the bright side of everything. May all beings be healed. May all beings be at peace. May God's will be done.

About the Author

Vimala McClure lives and writes from her home in the Ozarks of southern Missouri with her husband, three teenage children, two cats and an assortment of wildlife. She is the author of several books and the founder of the International Association of Infant Massage Instructors. Vimala has practiced meditation and yoga for over twenty years.

Enjoy these other fine books from NUCLEUS Publications!

Beyond the Superconscious Mind
Ananda Mitra $6.00 80pp. Order BS600
Based on yoga philosophy, this illuminating book explores both eastern and western understanding of how the mind works, including desire, recollection and reflection, intuition, paranormal phenomena, and meditation.

Some Still Want the Moon
A Woman's Introduction to Tantra Yoga
Vimala McClure $9.95 122pp. Order SM605
In a very personal way, McClure covers: breathing and relaxation, meditation and mantra, kundalini and chakras, yoga's creation theory, life changes such as menstruation, pregnancy, and menopause, and much more.

The Tao of Motherhood
Vimala McClure $10.95 176pp. Order TM225
"The Tao of Motherhood merges Eastern mysticism with Western practicality. Reading Vimala's book is like having Lao Tzu and Chuang Tzu in your living room holding your hand."
—Peggy O'Mara, editor and publisher, *Mothering Magazine*

The Vegetarian Lunchbasket
225 Easy, Nutritious Recipes for the Quality-Conscious Family on the Go
Linda Haynes $12.00 200pp. Order VL516
Try new ways of packing delicious lunches, using leftovers and combining foods. Use alternatives to meat and eggs, thus lowering fats and cholesterol without robbing yourself and your family of taste and variety.

Food for Thought
The Vegetarian Philosophy
Ananda Mitra $7.00 96pp. Order FT304
An excellent resource for beginning and established vegetarians, it covers all the reasons why a vegetarian diet is the most suitable for human beings and shows where to find the nutrients that compose a balanced, healthy vegetarian diet.

Order by phone toll free 1-800-762-6595
To order by mail please add $3.00 shipping & handling to price of first book ordered plus $.50 for each additional book, and send to:
NUCLEUS Publications, Rt 2 Box 49, Willow Springs MO 65793